THE SCREECH OWLS
OF BREAST CANCER

THE SCREECH OWLS OF BREAST CANCER

*How the demographic social and medical ill omens
highlighted by breast cancer are being ignored*

EUGENE G BREEN

authorHOUSE®

AuthorHouse™ UK Ltd.
1663 Liberty Drive
Bloomington, IN 47403 USA
www.authorhouse.co.uk
Phone: 0800.197.4150

Published by AuthorHouse   11/16/2013

ISBN: 978-1-4918-8280-1 (sc)
ISBN: 978-1-4918-8281-8 (e)

CONTENTS

Other works:

The Human Mind and Belief II—Unplugged

The Human Mind and Belief—Published September 2013

EXECUTIVE SUMMARY

This book is mainly about the 50% or more women who get breast cancer and who should not be getting it. It is about seeing why the incidence of breast cancer is way above "normal levels", and why cancer levels are twice as high in young women compared to young men. This is not an ordinary cancer. It has demographic, social, and philosophical tentacles and the casualties this year alone, number 1.6 million women with breast cancer. The answer as such is not just simply medical, but social and political as well.

This is in essence an investigative journalist type of "no frills" dissection, both clinical and forensic, of the story of breast cancer, and of why a dominant cause for it has not been found and eradicated. It spans medical, social and political aspects of the illness. It is a provocative journey through a potential minefield and compares the breast cancer story to those of the recent financial recession, the cigarette wars and the seminal steps of the specialty of epidemiology. The psychological flavour of the Pink Ribbon campaigns are delineated in broad strokes and the areas of birth control and demography are referred to as relevant ingredients in the story. The book is aimed at the intelligent lay and medical/paramedical reader and tries to stimulate appropriate reaction and to guide further personal study of the topic. This is needed to stem the tide of this awful cancer.

It is suggested that not everyone is singing from the same hymn sheet. The overall ideas expressed point to what could be seen as a serious failure in tackling this epidemic of breast cancer. The enormous numbers affected by it, the deaths and morbidity associated with it, and the growing numbers of young women getting aggressive breast cancer, all indicate a growing problem. Why this is so after 50 years of research and study and funding is bizarre.

The research presented is not a comprehensive tabulation of all the evidence to date. Others have done this and have added to the data on breast cancer. The evidence here is very recent in some cases and illustrative in others and these help to drive home various points. The discourse is at times outrageous or flighty, and this is done to emphasize points, to highlight contrasts and to refresh the reader's attention. They also are used to encourage the reader to not see breast cancer as a purely medical issue.

Whilst writing these pages one cannot but be all too aware of the thousands of women and their families who have suffered severely from this terrible cancer. One also is reminded and edified by all those generous people who do Pink Ribbon or other sponsored events and who fundraise. These are the unsung heroes of this illness. The researchers and doctors and pharmacists who advance the genuine cause of breast cancer are also to be praised. These people will I hope excuse any over exuberance or comments which are not meant to offend, but on the contrary are employed to act as a catalyst to flush out the truth.

The conclusion is that breast cancer is on the increase, and all the research and funding and doctors cannot solve it because they have been trying for 50 years and its spread and aggression is getting worse instead of better. Another focus is needed and information that is transparent and simple and accessible to all needs to be uncovered and needs to pin point the real cause for the excess breast cancer incidence.

The initial chapters are descriptive and set the scene. Later chapters contain referenced sources and point the way to further reading. Evidence to support the claims and overview contained in the initial chapters is presented later in the text.

There is also a focus on the softer evidence based societal reaction to breast cancer and the medical and political responses to it. This is done to highlight the big picture and to enable a clinical non biased eye to assess the story and make a judgement as to the real truth behind it. This is a crucial aspect of the study of breast cancer since it points to how and why we have arrived at where we are today. It uses other debacles like the Mid Staffordshire Hospital Report in UK, the 50 year delay in confirming cigarettes as the major cause of lung cancer and early death, and examples from the world of sport, to show how such mistakes and disasters occur. The answer is a mixture of deception, ignorance, and global blindness by both experts and ordinary people. These considerations also indicate where it will continue to go unless something is done to stop it.

The author is a psychiatrist with internal medicine experience and training and uses both the medical and psychiatric lenses to look at the societal and psychological aspects of the illness and also the scientific aetiological and epidemiological aspects. This broad view helps to see both the wood and the trees and therefore not to miss the big data by being too attentive to slight advances in specialized areas. The overall emphasis is on big data—population trends; societal reactions; raw cancer data in national/international data bases; new trends of the cancer etc. The media and internet roles are also highlighted. The forecast for breast cancer is getting worse, and unless something is done to root out the dominant cause especially in young women, the future is bleak. The book needs to be read in its totality because the initial chapters are only understandable in the light of the rest of the book which is less racy and more evidence based.

DISCLAIMER AND DECLARATION OF MOTIVATION

Why would anyone want to write a book about the causation of breast cancer? The answer is possibly because it is so common and it causes such devastation to so many women, many of whom are very young. Any insight therefore that throws some light on this plague has to be a very good thing. It also comes from an ethical imperative to say what you genuinely think is true, needs to be said, despite being so roundly denied and ignored, and constitutes a serious matter. What for example led the parents of Lorenzo to follow their passion in the now famous film "Lorenzo's Oil" and to achieve the impossible, finding a cure for his rare illness? What also leads people to attempt feats that stretch endurance to the limit like climbing Everest from the north face or swimming the 7 straits or doing a super ironman or discovering the cause for an illness? People become fired by a passion to achieve, or by a hunch about something, or experience "a worm that doesn't die" squirming away inside until it is expelled.

Sometimes it can be like having a thorn in your finger that hurts when you press and you aren't happy until you get it out. The thought that breast cancer is not all it is purported to be, and that a major cause or contributor is being forgotten about or not highlighted enough is a spur to shout this out and to probe further. The literature is absolutely overflowing with articles about breast cancer and they range from the scientific and medical to more lightweight websites. It is an army in full march with banners and trumpets and you could say where is it going or who is the enemy? Many think the enemy is behind the advancing line continuing to cause havoc and hiding completely protected by camouflage and even with the connivance of the generals! I'm talking about female hormones prescribed as oral contraceptives (OCs) and hormonal replacement therapy (HRT). These are much bigger players in the genesis of breast cancer than the official data on medication side effects leaflets, established cancer websites and pronouncements from medical bodies admit to. This is the issue at hand.

People who live with illness also achieve mammoth feats and they don't get to go on TV and nobody writes a book about them. Their parents and relatives also live heroic lives and sometimes it is harder to live with a sick person (for example depression) than to have it oneself. These are the unsung heroes we don't hear about. Breast cancer is one of the scourges of modern society, and many heroines and their relatives suffer in silence. Some however are not content to stay quiet and their very visual presence on the streets and at public events and in the media with the Pink Ribbon, shows that they are unhappy and are turning over every stone to try and bring this plague to an end.

So why write about breast cancer causation? The very visual image of Pink demonstration attracts attention. Being a doctor and having treated cancer, and knowing something about its cause and effects alerts one to the size of the Pink Ribbon campaign and gets one to focus in with special attention. Having personal experience of friends in their thirties who contracted breast cancer and suffered the treatments and anxiety and depression has had its impact. Hearing and seeing young women in their prime struck down by breast cancer pushes one to ask oneself "is this normal?" The intellectual curiosity and hunch that all is not right in world of breast cancer, that this is not a normal cancer behaviour pattern, forces one to investigate further and to challenge the standard dogma and explanations about the causes of breast cancer trotted out by all in sundry.

The frustration at seeing yet another breast-check clinic, or Pink Ribbon shop, or advertisement on a bill board with a young smiling woman for private insurance that will get you into—wait for it—eight cancer centres of excellence! Where am I? How about a ticket to eight saunas or bus tours, but eight super duper cancer clinics . . . just try and stop me! This has to be sick. This has to be OTT. This has to be wrong. You don't see advertisements for cancer centres for young men or dogs. Men's advertisements are for beer and is it now the case that women's advertisements are for cancer clinics? These reasons plus the hibernation of the medical literature on producing any fresh new insights into the aetiology of breast cancer stimulates one to want to get an answer. The medical literature yawns with user fatigue about the cause of breast cancer as it reports another bland unconvincing metanalysis or statistical take on why (OCs) and (HRT) do not really cause much breast cancer.

This is what confronts us on a daily basis. Maybe everyone knows why breast cancer is so common and are saying nothing. Maybe the women know and let on they don't. Maybe they are not prepared to stop the pills and HRT and nip it in the bud. Much like a guy smoking and the doctor says "unless you stop smoking you are going to die" and he says "ok doc I'll take me chances". Maybe that is what all the hype and sponsored marathons and coffee mornings are about—therapy sessions for people doing the wrong thing and wanting solace and catharsis or relief because they know its wrong; or for people mixed up and not willing to find out the truth. The women know or don't want to know that HRT and OCs cause breast cancer because they just want to take their chances and live as they want. Taking that to be the case why all the hype and publicity and why the shouting? (Pink Ribbon events, web sites, slogans, bumper stickers . . . .). The alcoholic knows he will get cirrhosis, and the diabetic knows he can't eat sugars but there are no bill boards or purple or mauve ribbons. There is no fashion shop for cirrhosis shirts or diabetic ties. They are the great unwashed they are getting their comeuppances and they know it and they are responsible, so no crowing or complaining but "just do what you can doc". Not so with breast cancer. TV shows and DJs and parties and pink everything. Why? Why not suffer quietly like the rest of the sick? Why not "do what you can doc" and leave it like that? But no sir!

This tells us it is not all it is cooked up to be. This is not a normal human reaction. Most women with one illness or another are like your chronic bronchitic or cirrhotic they get on with it and do their best without fanfare or razzmatazz. Why not with breast cancer folk? Is it because they are struck down so young? Is it because there are so many? Is it because it has taken so long to get the answer to its cause? Is it because they are frustrated because the golden egg is rotten after all? The gilded pill is in fact poisonous. That is what could be driving the hysteria. That would explain the decibel level around breast cancer.

Maybe that is the motivation behind writing. The unusual hype around breast cancer is unusual and unprecedented and it is not normal. It is sustained and growing and vociferous. These could be characteristics of even anger and frustration. The public fund raisers and pink merchandise do draw attention to the issue, and whereas the majority of promoters of the breast cancer cause are not strident there definitely seems to be an edge to it. A very average person would have no problem pointing to the pill and HRT as a major cause of breast cancer when given the data. The answer is plain and simple and is there for the asking. The doctors and scientists could easily be asked to recall, reconsider, and reassess the safety profile of the pill and HRT. This was never done. It needs to be done. It is the only way to solve both the issue of breast cancer numbers and also the anger and reaction around it.

If this is the case why are all the experts and doctors not saying it? The truth is that many doctors and scientists have been pointing this out for years but are being ignored and the limelight been given to those that say the opposite. Chris Kahlenborn describes this pattern in his book which will be seen later. Also this type of behaviour is not uncommon. Take the recent financial recession. Look at Bernie Madoff's ponzie scheme or Lehman Brothers. Who said what when? No one said anything and that is why the world is in recession. The regulators are now sifting through the financial debris and eventually heads are rolling and companies and banks and enterprises are folding. Fannie Mae and Freddie Mac were similarly insolvent and the repossessionists are now boarding up houses and people are in serious distress. This calamity could have been prevented in many countries and institutions if those at the top were awake to what was happening. The Costa Concordia would not have gone aground if the captain was in control. Fatal negligence and delusional type thinking at the highest level does and has caused shipwreck for many.

Another way to understand this type of mind set is to look at the flat earth crew and Galileo. What a thing to say that the earth circled the sun sure everyone knows the sun circles the earth! Or that bacteria cause peptic ulcers, and now every one with an ulcer gets a course of 3 antibiotics. Or that women and men would travel to the moon? The point is that accepted dogma is as good as its genuine challenge and clarity and honesty and transparency do win out. To come close to home there have been many retractions in the medical literature over the years and even this week we see that tens of thousands of deaths may have been caused by using beta blockers during surgery. The Liverpool Care Pathway beloved by the NHS and NICE in UK recently was closed due to gross malpractice. So, errors do abound. The more accepted and embedded the dogma the harder they are to debunk but the big picture and honest appraisal uncover the flaws. Most medical journals now have a section called "errata" for mistakes in previous editions. This is business as usual and undoubtedly mistakes of these and greater magnitudes will continue to occur due to human error.

It is not accepted by the medical establishment that the pill is a major cause of breast cancer. The key journals and opinion leaders grudgingly accept that OCs and HRT may play some small part in breast cancer causation but no more than that. There are however many straws in the wind indicating that the laws of nature are unclear in this case i.e. the really dominant cause of breast cancer.

Firstly, cancer is usually a disease of older people. Breast cancer affects a very large number of young women compared with any other cancer in either sex. The population trends are freely available in Cancer Research UK or SEER in USA or EUCAN the European Cancer Observatory and they confirm more than double the numbers of young women getting cancer compared to men of the same ages. This is predominantly breast cancer in the women.

Secondly, cancer in young mammals to the extent it is seen in women does not happen.

Thirdly when a disease breaks standard parameters like levels of incidence a cause is sought and after a reasonable amount of time one is found. This has not occurred after 50 years or more of breast cancer research. This is bizarre.

Fourthly, breast cancer is spreading now to underdeveloped countries along with the spread of OCs pointing to an obvious connection.

Fifthly, the mass screening for breast cancer has clouded the picture more by allowing people to say "oh it is increasing because we are now picking it up much better and earlier than we did before". This is untrue because the patterns were already well established before the screening started and also in places where there is no screening the incidence is high.

Sixthly, with all the research the incidence is not dropping but is actually getting more common showing that the cause is still there and even propagating further. Why have the levels of breast cancer not dropped in 35 years? The answer is because the cause has been missed and it is still active. Eradicate the cause and the numbers with breast cancer would plummet. This happened with HRT in Canada and USA when it was stopped and the results were that levels of breast cancer plummeted. The very same would occur with the pill. Stop it and breast cancer will drop to levels of any cancer in the appropriate age group.

This must be known by all, but why it is an open secret and no one opens the lid on this Pandora's Box? Who knows? Have the drug companies got data on file showing gross effects on breast tissue that are possibly in old archives? This would not be unusual. Drug companies are often investigated for data issues. Glaxo Smith Kline was fined 3 billion dollars last year for inappropriate sales practice and withholding safety data. The new diabetic drugs and the arthritic drugs are more recent casualties with Vioxx being taken off the shelves due to heart attack data being fudged. Could the OC and HRT researchers have good data on file somewhere which would throw light on the breast cancer OC/HRT connection?

These factors all present a scenario in the OC world ripe for exploitation by anyone with a reason to promote their use and sales regardless of health and safety concerns. The relatively unregulated development and emergence and propagation of female hormone medications and their meteoric rise in use present a picture of the horse being long gone before the stable door was closed, and strict accountable health and safety checks put in place. The scene in 1960 with the launch of OCs was set for either a tremendous discovery with the immediate and cost free liberation of women from child rearing and house duties thanks to a new little pill; or an aftermath after the excitement and joy had quietened to the sober reality of a new plague that just won't abate or go away. The latter unfortunately has visited millions of young women and not only in the shape of breast cancer but also with blood clots, strokes and pulmonary emboli to mention a few adverse reactions. One wonders how a drug with such a harrowing track record is still on the market.

THE SCANDAL OF BREAST CANCER

Setting the scene

What has happened in the past 50 years to explain the ravages of breast cancer? Why are young women dying or living in fear of contracting the deadly illness? Why women? Why not men or other mammals? Why is this illness visited on women in their prime? This is the reality and a scan of pink merchandise and shops and sponsored runs etc. show how widespread is the spread of breast cancer.

Scientists and doctors and social commentators all probe and investigate and research the nature of breast cancer, how it grows and what countries have it most. The spotlight is now (and has been for at least 50 years) on its metabolism, it's receptors and its treatment, but causation is down the scale as regards public or professional attention. This "why?" question has been bypassed to a certain extent and yet it is the most important aspect of the illness. The tanks have advanced and meantime the enemy is firmly entrenched behind the advancing line happy to keep jeopardizing the success of the battle at will. This is proven by the fact that despite all the effort being expended on researching breast cancer it still continues to spread and increase in aggression.

A very significant at issue is that the cancer in question, breast cancer, is predominantly hormone (oestrogen and progesterone) dependent, driven and ignited. The medical treatment is to reduce hormone exposure with anti-oestrogen drugs. The rise in breast cancer incidence parallels and mirrors the rise in the use of female hormones either used as contraceptive pills or as HRT (menopausal hormone replacement therapy). This is mapped by time across decades—the more use of pills or HRT the more breast cancer; and geography, countries using more hormones get more breast cancer. These are facts like the weather satellite picture which shows where the clouds are, this breast cancer satellite picture is freely available to all on SEER statistics (USA) and statistics of cancer incidence from most if not all developed countries.

Broad picture

The reality and truth of the situation is there for all to see. Look at the rising numbers with breast cancer. Look at the rising use of female hormones. Look at the pattern of spread of breast cancer from developed world to third world after introduction of the pill. Look at men or animals and there is no similar pattern of cancer either of breast cancer in female animals or of prostate or other cancer in young men. Look at female dogs that are spayed (castrated) before first heat and they very rarely if ever get breast cancer (because the source of female hormones is gone) whereas unspayed female dogs do. Look at lung cancer which was also of vast proportions and the scientific community confirmed the obvious—that cigarettes were the culprit. Look at skin cancer and its relationship to UV light exposure. Look at bowel cancer and its relationship to western constipating diets. They are all simple in the sense that what is obvious is true. They also have similar satellite pictures to breast cancer across time and geography. The rise of cigarette smoking tallied with the rise of lung cancer. The rise of refined western diets corresponded to the rise of bowel cancer. To some extent science is simple, you look at the obvious and often you are right. This is the evidence in theses common cancers.

What then is obvious about the possible cause of breast cancer? It's the hormones. Take out the hormones and like the spayed bitches you don't get breast cancer. (Not to the same extent). There are multiple generic causes of cancer ranging from genetic predisposition, to friction, to carcinogen exposure in food, inhalants (cigarettes), UV light, obesity and so on. The IARC institution (International Agency for Research on Cancer) has a list of such carcinogens for those interested. There are other cancer provoking agents like invisible radon gas in houses, radiation, even alcohol and all told each human body gets its fair share of carcinogen exposure each day, but these atmospheric or environmental carcinogens should not pick out women, no more than lungs or bowels, and so there must be a female reason for breast cancer. What are women exposed to that animals or men are not? It is female hormones in the pill or HRT.

The picture is not easy on one hand and very easy on the other. Reliable records and transparent data are necessary to see what numbers were affected in let's say 1945, 1960, and 1980 and so on. What the sales or exposure to pills or HRT were for corresponding years and in what countries. What women took what hormone for how long? This isn't complicated science but the scientific literature that publishes these studies is anything but clear. That's the problem. There are contradictory studies and millions of women have been studied and still there isn't a true vision of the causation of the problem.

Official websites for cancer in USA, UK, and Canada to mention a few all say that the pill confers a slight risk of breast cancer. The IARC institute classifies the contraceptive pill as a carcinogen. Once you have a collection of cancer inducing agents together you get an added or cumulative exposure to cancer risk. Let's say you have obesity and alcohol and cigarettes well then you are at risk. Take extra female hormones on top of this and the stakes are really high for cancer. That's not all. You may even succumb before the cancer has had a chance to raise its head by a blood clot to the brain or lung, which again is well described with the pill, HRT and obesity.

Drug surveillance

All drugs that reach the market are now rigorously tested for safety in animals first and then in humans. After what are called phase three trials and a clean bill of health they are then released on the public and are subject to post marketing surveillance. Many block buster drugs have been removed from circulation recently in this process. The cox 2 inhibitors such as Vioxx were withdrawn, and the new diabetic drugs are under close monitoring at present for adverse side effects. It costs 5 to 10 hundred million dollars to bring a new drug to the shop shelf. That is a colossal amount of money and work. The pressures to minimize any side effects that may hamper a drug's launch are therefore great. The number of studies that show "no", or "a poor effect" of a drug, are often multiples of those that show a "beneficial effect" but only the "good result" ones get to be published and marketed. This is legal until now but obviously opaque practice. A new block buster drug like Lipostat is worth billions of dollars. The possibility of such a product going to market with the billions of dollars in sales easily clouds everything else especially when it is in later phase trials. That is why vigilance and impartiality are paramount in this business. That is why the FDA and European drug surveillance and monitoring bodies exist. These independent watchdogs patrol the drug world and should and do prevent dangerous products reaching the public.

The "good news" for the pill and its backers was that the horse had already bolted before the proper drug trials were done. OCs never had rigorous animal or human trials that were independently assessed. The push for a pill that would control fertility was so powerful that all dissenting or health and safety voices were steamrolled on its way to the market. The FDA approved the pill for contraceptive purposes in 1960 and it is widely accepted that the focus was so powerfully on its contraceptive effect that the adverse effect profile was played down or ignored. It was 10 years before the increase in clots was established and the breast cancer risk is even today disputed.

What the experts say

The usual comment by all health establishments or cancer institutes about OCs is that they confer a slight or small risk of causing breast cancer; however they add that this risk is counteracted by its reduction of cancer of the womb. If this is all true why is there such hype and attention and breast screening? Why is the female population subject to scans and even prophylactic mastectomy, as Angeline Jolly recently had? If it is a non event well then let the pink band wagon disappear and resume life as usual. This Pink Ribbon is an "in your face publicity" world wide (developed world) around breast cancer. Why? Is it a publicity stunt? Is it a smoke screen for something else? Or is it because "the song remembers when" i.e. the words and opinions all say one thing but the stark raving reality is that "I lost my breast and Mary did and poor Clare died at 37". Ooops! . . . . some thing is wrong. The windows are blowing in, the slates are coming down the trees are uprooted and the weather man says there are slight risks of gusty weather. There is a disconnect between the diplomacy of medical institutions, pill information leaflets, women's magazines and women in distress. The narrative of world health on satellite view is that the women are hurting; they are saying it, their husbands and children are out in sympathy and no receding in the ravages of breast cancer has occurred in over 50 years. They are being headed off at the pass and instead of sitting down with the women and coming clean or being open to what they are saying, the response is to keep the blinkers on and siphon all the money into treatment.

Meantime Melinda Gates in all her wisdom has donated billions to meet "the unmet contraceptive needs of the third world" by supplying pills. To understand the drama unfolding we see on the one hand millions of women publicly demonstrating solidarity and support for breast cancer sufferers and survivors, and on the other hand an absolute denial, ignoring or hiding of the even remote possibility that pills, HRT and breast cancer could be more closely connected by the donation of millions to the promotion of OCs. This calls for a recall and a recount or a reassessment at least. When Toyota who "build the best cars in the world" as the advertisement says had a problem with the new Prius all the world wide Prius models were recalled and checked. The women of the world are shouting "hey we are fed up of this breast cancer and the screening and the early deaths and the mastectomies. Do you not hear us? We are the ones decked out in Pink with the logos on our cars". Yes the message is loud and clear. It is like a football crowd shouting "Free Ref" and the referee ignores them and the game carries on. Why does not someone with authority press the pause button and say "What is this all about? Is this worse than the experts tell us or have the women all gone crazy?" Let's look at it. Is breast cancer way out of control is question one. Question two is why, and question three is what do we do about it?

The answer to 1 is yes. The answer to question 2 is the pill and HRT. The answer to question 3 is stop giving them out until it is all checked out. What is the definitive study? Ideally you should have 1000 women on the pill for 10 to 20 years and a similar number not on the pill for the same duration and compare cancer in one group with that in the other. This should by rights be at least a 40 or 50 year study because the cancer may not show until later. This has not been done transparently and successfully without the involvement of vested interests. There have been studies that seem reputable that have shown 30 to 35 per cent increases in breast cancer due to pill exposure but these are negated by other ones that don't show any increase.

The key studies

The water-shed studies are what are called meta-analyses. These are statistical methods similar to a smoothie machine. You put apples and peaches and oranges and fruit juice in and whirl them all together and you get a delicious fruity drink. So you establish criteria for research studies and pick those that fulfil the ground rules you make, and whirl them all together with complex statistical software and you get an amorphous product with a little of everything. The good and bad are admixed and neutrality rules OK. This is a little unfair because when properly and transparently done these are good tools but the margin for error and obfuscation are significant. So if you put squeaky clean data in with dirty data you cancel the good stuff with the murky stuff and the truth is missed for the sake of compromise or full inclusion, but this is bad science and flawed logic. When you mix data showing large cancer effects with OCs and HRT with data showing little effect both cancel each other out. They cannot be both right and therefore the answer is to conduct simple well powered and unbiased, independently funded studies and see what they show.

An analysis of every research paper that went into the water-shed metanalysis papers would be required and the thoroughness and transparency of the raw data inspected. This is impossible at this late stage. Comprehensive mammal studies are also required. They should be independently conducted to prevent interference or contamination by interested parties. Meticulous attention to technique and planning combined with documentation of timing of exposure to female hormones would be obligatory. These parameters would need to be decided by expert veterinarians and the subsequent examining of breast tissue be done by vets who did not know what animals got what feed. This has not been done or if it was done the results are not published. This is a basic requirement for the approval of any drug. It was not done for the pill. It needs to be done and published. The literature as it stands is anything but clear. There are reputable centres showing large increases in cancer due to the OCs and these need to be confirmed or denied by reputable replication without vested interest (any lobby) involvement. If this does not happen the scourge of breast cancer will continue because a cause has not been found.

Causation of cancer

Causation in medicine is all important. When a cause for a condition is identified a definitive cure can be tackled. When a cause is not found treatment focuses on relieving the symptoms and some times a serendipitous cure is found and no one can say how it works. Penicillin was an example that worked and later why it worked was found out. The genetics and causation of cancer per se is extraordinarily well researched and new treatments for many cancers have been developed and discovered. This is great news. A cure for breast cancer may also be found and advances are being made with anti-oestrogens and surgeries and radiotherapy. Better if it never happened in the first place and prevention is always better than cure. Prevention of breast cancer is what is at stake and all of the data about spread, ages affected, and comparisons to other cancers suggest a key cause has not been identified. This is remarkable given the long time of at least 50 years that it is being researched. Most illnesses are understood in much less time. AIDS took 6 years from the first documented case in New York in 1981 to the isolation of the virus in 1986. Bowel cancer and diet connection has been established for decades now. The lung cancer cigarette controversy took much too long 50 years plus and there was a key reason for this which we will see below. With the thousands of researchers and billions of dollars gone into breast cancer research it seems that there must be something radically wrong, since it is increasing in western countries and spreading to new areas.

Cigarettes and cancer

The cigarette lung cancer story may be indicative of what can hamper discovery of a serious cause of illness when vested interests are involved. In 1994 the heads of the major US tobacco companies testified before Congress: (1) that the evidence that cigarettes caused cancer and heart disease was inconclusive; (2) that cigarettes were not addictive and; (3) that they did not market to children. Approximately 4 weeks later data from company archives clearly showed that tobacco companies knew for decades that cigarettes caused early deaths, were addictive and that their programme to support scientific research on smoking and health was a sham. The subsequent revelation of cover up and lies and scientific fraud is well documented. The latest battle was with "low tar brands" which were touted as being safer but in reality are worse because they are inhaled more deeply. The sub headings in a review of the history of tobacco and cancer by Michael Cummings et al (in 2007 issue of Cancer Epidemiology Biomarkers and Prevention), is instructive and revealing. They go;

"Smoking causes cancer: When did they know?" (The answer is that they knew all along).

"Conspiracy to deceive" This confirms that the tobacco industry conspired to make false, deceptive and misleading public statements about cigarettes from 1954. Advertisements were published questioning research reporting smoking as a cause of cancer, endorsing the safety of their brands of cigarettes and donating serious funds to research the allegations that smoking was injurious to health. These advertisements were put into 448 newspapers and would have been seen by 43 million people.

"Science for Sale". This catalogues the mercenary scientific community who lied through their teeth to protect their sponsor the tobacco industry, and in so doing paraded as the wolf in sheep's clothing delaying the publication of ill health effects from smoking for decades. The usual ploys were used "the data is controversial we will have to do more research . . . ."

"Have Tobacco Companies Changed?" The short answer is no.

Bias

Sometimes it is the big picture that tells the story and missing the wood for the trees is a common error. Bias is powerful and it clouds thinking. When you don't want something to be true almost nothing will convince you otherwise. Take an example. Depending on how much you love your son and want him to be innocent, you hope against hope that he is OK, until you are confronted by the facts or incontrovertible evidence that he did kill someone or whatever. Even then you make excuses and maybe don't accept it. This is similar to the euphoria and liberation and overwhelming reaction to the pill and its life changing potential that occurred on its discovery, and most didn't want to hear anything bad about it and still don't.

Here we then have a wolf in sheep's clothing smiling all its way to new countries and populations in the underdeveloped world. Meantime any talk of increase in breast cancer or blood clots are air brushed from publicity by experts denying it, and by certain medical establishments contradicting it, referencing milestone research papers that "show beyond all doubt that the pill is safe". A crime writer should be writing this.

Yes the medical literature is contradictory and that is the root cause for the ongoing failure to arrest this cancer epidemic. The latest sales pitch goes something like: "we have moved on and the new pills are much safer than the older ones and have much less oestrogen." . . . . I wonder why less oestrogen? (Sounds like much less tar in cigarettes revisited?) Why less oestrogen? Is it to reduce bloating, ankle swelling, tenderness in breast tissue, less clots and also less hormonal assault on breast cells?

Physiology

What happens to healthy women as regards hormones? Healthy women have cycles that are reflected in hormonal peaks and troughs that in their turn switch on and off ovulation every month. This pattern continues from menarche to menopause. What happens when you take the pill? The synthetic oestrogen and progesterone take over and prevent transmitter release from the pituitary and so stop ovulation. This said in another way is that there is a constant high of female hormones instead of peaks and troughs and the body is taking a bigger hormone hit including of course the breast. This constitutes a risk for any female hormone dependent tumour and hence the risk of more breast cancer. This is simple and transparent and obvious like cigarettes and lungs and food and the gut. The wrong stuff in a regular way to an organ and it malfunctions and cancer develops in some. Stop the noxious exposure and the risk declines. The breast is a gland that has the function of producing milk under control of hormones. The cells are hormone sensitive. The way to get at the breast is by the blood stream since it is a closed organ, and the agent to use is something the breast cells will absorb and process, and therefore something that gets into the DNA and cell replication cycle. This is where cancer grows—at cell replication, and any speed up slow down or interference will cause malfunction and cancer risk. Hormones get right into the cell DNA and replication process and therefore too much hormone over stimulates the cells leading to cancer.

This is a very simplified account of what happens and why hormones are exactly what you don't need as regards getting breast cancer.

The most recent edition of Annals of Internal Medicine confirms this with their article: "Medications for risk reduction of primary breast cancer in women: Preventive Services Task Force Recommendation Statement" by V. Moyer et al. Sept 2013. They issue recommendations for use of tamoxifen and raloxifene in women at high risk of breast cancer. They note that these anti-oestrogen medications do confer some protection especially in oestrogen positive sensitive tumours. The interesting thing about this statement and the BCRA breast cancer risk assessor (a recognised assessment tool for breast cancer) is that female hormone exposure (OCs and HRT) are again in the back rows of risk factors and don't feature as such compared to genetics, family history and prior history. These latter are crucial in this particular cancer group, but female hormones are also crucial and they are not even mentioned in the National Cancer Risk Assessment Tool. The point that this article confirms is that oestrogen and cancer are very much connected.

BREAST CANCER BLINDNESS

Why all the convulsions and societal upheaval due to breast cancer? Why all the chat shows and survivor pressure groups and breast cancer days? Why the unrest and dysphoria in the female population due to breast cancer? Why the lack of peace and acceptance and calm around the entire issue? When was the last time such widespread uneasiness occurred in society? People usually behave in this way when they are upset and want their rights back, for example. People take to the street when they are energized by an injustice. Marches for workers rights, marches for less taxes, marches for social injustice and so on. When was the last time there was a mass demonstration for celiac disease or obesity or lung cancer? Never? Why for breast cancer? Is there more of a social rights flavour to it or have women's rights been infringed?

The answer has to be yes. It is the only way to explain and understand the ongoing and widespread demonstration about breast cancer. Women are hurting and they want people to sit up and pay attention and do something about it. The female population is up in arms and they don't know where to direct their anger and so we see public demonstrations of every sort. What would calm the situation and bring peace back to these suffering people? The answer is clear transparent and truthful answers to their plight. The answer is to tell them what is going on. They have been tormented; they cannot finger the culprit but this they do know that they are being targeted. This is the swirling distressing feeling that won't go away because it is being stoked and fanned by ever more new cases of breast cancer and it just seems to go on and on.

Ok sit down and see what is happening, where it is happening, who should know why it is still happening after 50 years and then pause. What emerges is that the breast cancer epidemic is not abating and in fact in some circles it is getting worse (black Americans, third world, first world, young females). It should be abating with all the screening and chemotherapy and ancillary data about keeping weight down, and taking fish oils and avoiding cigarettes and fatty diets. It is not however. The very same would happen with cervical cancer if all these measures were taken and the wolf in sheep's clothing was missed. For cervical cancer this wolf is promiscuity—multiple sexual partners. So the sweet spot again is not environmental (inhalants, UV light, radon . . . .) but the obvious: cervix and cancer and what touches or hits the cervix? Yes sexual activity. The same applies in a similar way to lung cancer. Remove all the obesity and alcohol, and fatty diets and the lung cancer epidemic roars on. The timid little wolf of course is the cigarette. Very obvious and yet it took 50 years to confirm. Now answer yourself, what about breast cancer what is the wolf in sheep's clothing?

What is the obvious answer? Why is it the obvious answer? Why is no one saying it? The answer is female hormones either as the pill or as HRT. It is obvious because they zone right in on breast tissue, like cigarettes and lungs or food and bowel. Nobody is saying it because those that do are ignored and everyone is referred to the medical evidence which as mentioned above is contradictory.

The downside of this is the cancer that comes from too much hormones for too long. Too much of anything is bad for you the adage says and this certainly applies to hormones. Too much growth hormone for endurance sports gives you blood pressure and heart attacks. Too much steroid for sport also gives heart problems—Flo Jo comes to mind, and too much cortisol give obesity and diabetes. They all cause early death. The keep-fit gyms that abuse creatine and anabolic steroids are stoking hypercholesterolemia and hypertension and cardiovascular problems for their users. The evidence is well documented.

If you google hyper-estrogenemia or too much oestrogen, you are confronted by acres of data on awful side effects of too much oestrogen including breast cancer. In fact 80% of breast cancers are oestrogen dependent or driven so extra hormones (OCs, HRT) should be contra-indicated in most women. The sad thing is that when you google oestrogen in one form or another you find prime sites advertising "how to lower your oestrogen level" and "how I eat my way to lower oestrogen" type of material. The first question to ask is: why lower it? What's the idea? On the contrary maybe I will be more attractive if I increase my oestrogen one might think. But no these sites tell you that everything is full of oestrogen—white coating on drink cans and bottles, nail varnish, some foods, adipose tissue and some really good ones . . . like toiletries, pesticides, preservatives . . . These are touted but absolutely never ever a word about shovelling in oestrogen by the spoonful in pills and HRT. This is really strange.

The point at issue being that if you take extra oestrogen 5 or 7 days a week what do you get but hyper oestrogenemia all of the time, and this is a time-bomb waiting to get either the breast or some other system? This is definite. There are acute hyper oestrogenemic states usually caused by stimulants of ovulation in the IVF situation. These raise oestrogen and the clinical results are worth looking up. They include bloating, going on to critical health issues.

SORRY—EUREKA MOMENT

When you look up the Cancer Research UK website you get some very good data. What it says is that the incidence of any cancer per year in UK in women aged 25 to 49 is 25500 compared to 11000 in males of the same age bracket. The high female figures are due to the high levels of breast cancer. This site states clearly that young women get more than twice the amount of cancer that males get. It also confirms that breast cancer is the most common cancer of all cancers with 50,000 cases in 2010. It states that HRT increases the risk of breast cancer 66% and the pill by "a quarter" i.e. 25%. This is the first time such a definite figure has been used either for HRT or OCs in any official site and they certainly seem more realistic than heretofore. In "causes" it states for example that "current users of oral contraceptives have a quarter increase in risk of getting breast cancer but only 1% of breast cancer cases in UK each year are linked to oral contraceptives". (See Breast Cancer key facts and click causes in this site). It was never stated as much as a "quarter" before. It also says in another part of the site "the use of oral contraceptives increases the risk of breast cancer in current and recent users but there is no significant excess risk ten or more years after stopping use". This seems vaguer as regards risk and hides the true extent of the problem. Again, 25% is still very modest increase in risk of breast cancer from OCs compared to what some researchers report—40% plus, to be seen later.

Again one must ask why women get so much breast cancer since they are exposed to the same environment as males—that is, except for female hormone consumption. Does this mean that if women did not take the pill the cancer levels would drop to the male levels of 11,000 cases per year? The answer is why not? Yes. The excess of 14,500 breast cancer cases per year over the male numbers must be due to some toxin and this has to be the pill, since HRT is taken by older women. This is further supported by the finding that the incidence of breast cancer in England has increased almost 70% since the mid 1970s, without a seemingly identifiable cause. Also of note is that the incidence of breast cancer in UK has increased further by about 6% in the past ten years. Why is this? There must be a cause that is still being missed. The lifetime risk for breast cancer is now 1 in 8 for women in UK. These facts are very clearly stated in this website. They paint the stark picture of young women getting cancer early. The overall incidence of beast cancer per year is 50,000 and of these 25,500 are less than 49 years old i.e. 50%. This compares to bowel cancer where more than 60% of cases occur in people over 60 years of age. Breast cancer is therefore a cancer that affects women early in life. Lung cancer which affects 42,000 people every year and has a very well defined cause in cigarettes is the second most common cancer in UK, and it also hits people over 60 years of age with 80% being in this age group of new cases (same website).

The picture emerging from this 2013 web site is that breast cancer is by far the commonest cancer in young people of either sex. There is no cancer in males of 25 to 49 years with an incidence anywhere near that of breast cancer in women. This is a cause for concern. The HRT and OC incidence risk rate increases of 66% and 25% respectively have never been as openly published before and they agree in broad terms with the USA and Canadian HRT trials previously mentioned, and also with some reputable OC studies published to be seen later. This looks like a tentative admittance by a reputable site that there is more to female hormone exposure (HRT, OC) than small risk. It suggests that the message may be getting through and that a full "government health warning" may be a remote possibility just as occurred with cigarettes.

Breast cancer has been and is and will be an enormous epidemic that should have been stopped years ago. It is estimated that 1.6 million are affected with breast cancer worldwide at present. There are over 235,000 new cases each year in USA and no sign of abating. Similar websites from other countries show the same situation. There is marked variation in EU countries with some eastern countries with incidence less than half that in UK and France for example. In Greece 58 per 100,000 women and in Denmark 142 per 100,000 women got breast cancer in 2012. The variations may only add to the confusion and suffice it to say that UK is one of the worst affected by breast cancer in Europe.

This is the first web site or official cancer site seen by the author that put anything like a reasonable risk link to HRT and OCs. This is new. Most of the other official sites still quote the "slight risk" description. Other sites like The American Cancer Society also refer to increased risk in current users of OCs but do not get near the 25% figure the British site quotes. The breaking news about breast cancer aetiology from officialdom (cancer institutes, medical sites, national cancer sites) is that there is no news. There is a numbing glazed look at the statistics as they come in year on year slowly getting worse (6% increase breast cancer UK past 10 years) and like seeing a child slowly falling out of a pram the onlookers are distracted by other issues. The satellite picture of breast cancer is getting darker and unless female hormones are transparently and decisively outruled as the major cause acceptable to all to see then it must be concluded that they are the major cause of breast cancer. This is because they are the obvious one and have not been outruled clearly honestly and transparently and subsequently eradicated with an assessment of the effect of this on the incidence of breast cancer.

It must be acknowledged that the Cancer Research UK site is excellent and it puts the UK picture very clearly. It says the numbers and possibly for the first time puts figures on risk associated with various toxins including HRT and OCs. The OC warning is still weak and why say a "quarter" instead of 25% which is more eye catching? It is a start and American sites may follow suit in time. A 70% increase in incidence since 1970 and a further 6% increase in the last 10 years, and young women having over twice the cancer rates of young men (Cancer Research UK site) is a major health problem whose cause is still very active and spreading to new populations.

DEMOGRAPHY

The key argument used to prevent any reduction in the use of OCs is that of population explosion. The idea goes something like: "How will we feed all these people? We have seen the 7th billionth baby born this year and there is an exponential growth in population spiralling out of control. It must be stopped and the planet saved from all the green house gases these people are producing. The ice caps are melting, the ozone is disappearing, the sea is rising, the temperature is rising, and humans are to blame. Stop them reproducing". One child one family sounds familiar and the result is the skewing of the Chinese population towards a decline in female numbers.

There are a few questions about population. Has any other species overpopulated the planet? No. Why? What is the mammal population of the world and is it increasing or decreasing? Scientific American says there are 5,487 mammal species and that there are about 30 mice to every human. It further states that 1,700 scientists spent 5 years surveying the world's mammals and that 52% are declining in numbers. Animals do not use contraceptives and their numbers have not increased exponentially. They usually do not live as long as humans and a sudden peak in numbers could be easily wiped out with a cold snap or food shortage. Nature stabilises the environment and makes sure that biodiversity whether it involves animals or plants or microbes is maintained equitably.

When you search the Food and Agriculture Organisation of The United Nations website you get a world animal count. There are 6 billion horses, 11 billion asses, and 24 billion world livestock, between cattle and pigs and sheep etc. The mammals number 400 billion and fish over a trillion. Birds number 400 billion and amphibians, reptiles, insects zooplankton etc. makes an enormous figure dwarfing anything the human count of 7 billion comes near. There is world population exuberance and humans even if they number 7 billion are in the tiny minority. Humans are mammals and are definitely threatened with extinction at least in some countries. In Japan for example the percentage of the population over 65 years of age is 20% and rising. The same is happening in Europe and USA. At present the percentage of the European population over 65 years is 12 to 15% and this is rapidly rising. Natural wastage with death, illness, infertility, famine, war, and all the myriad of causes of early death wipe percentages of the world population in an ongoing way. The natural trend for any mammal is to decline in numbers as with the 5487 other species and only by conserving them do many survive extinction. Man is not a new species, he is not an artificially implanted species, and he was and is and will be a natural resident of earth and is a full member of earth's ecology. He has existed thousands of years and why is there now a population problem and—not one of decline or extinction but of over population? This seems bizarre and what could account for it if it were true? Better food supply, less illness, better living conditions would all help man to survive longer. Better maternity care and vaccination programmes undoubtedly contribute to preserving human life, but could all of these factors lead to overpopulation? Where have the natural checks and balances of nature gone? Why has this not happened until now? Nature is true to itself and corrects errors—freaks of nature do occur but are not sustained and of a level that would destabilise the entire ecosystem.

There are a definable number of animals and humans on the planet and a definable number of bugs and fish, and a definable quantity of oxygen and water and air and potential to produce food. Which of these is creaking at the seams? What life support on earth is under threat and why? Could the behaviour of tiny beings like humans jeopardise the planets homeostasis and cause the oceans to rise, the climate to change and the crops to fail? Yes, is the probable answer to this but it is not the numbers that matter but the behaviour. Several atomic bombs or neutron bombs would do untold damage to everything. Whether man is capable of blowing up the planet is for another day. Whether he can change weather by pumping out carbon or green house gases is a scientific question, but certainly the planet can house many trillions of humans provided they behave well and don't damage the ecosystem that sustains all life here. It is therefore not the population but what the population does. There is not a crisis in overpopulation but possibly in overproduction of noxious chemicals and gases and a handful of people could do this with the technology available today.

The world has changed and can now accommodate multiples of the population it once did because of the technology and ability to produce food for billions. The caveat is that they must not damage the environment. The only reason the human population is increasing unlike most if not all other species is because living conditions or the human environment has greatly improved, and can now sustain more people than ever thought imaginable. New rules must apply to powerful new technologies and the science that keeps abreast of development must inform human behaviour.

It does not make sense to contracept Europe and USA and end up with an elderly population supported by immigrants. The European environment cannot thrive and survive without young Europeans forming the labour market and supporting the aging population. Africa and India for example will continue to reproduce and die as they always did until development makes the human habitat more liveable in, and until it can support life for an average of 80 years instead of the present 50. (Most countries in Africa have life spans of 45 to 60 years). Each continent should be self sufficient in humans to stabilise growth and support the old and educate and feed the young. At present Africa, the Middle East and China among others are supporting the old men of Europe and USA and this is because of the pill. There are fewer kids in Europe or USA and these civilizations are passing on to other races because of a lack of indigenous populations.

The point is that nature follows set innate patterns and is equipped to cope with natural ecological swings and fluxes. By interfering artificially with it by widespread birth control problems arise. Nature looks after animals and plants and if we behave as humans should behave nature will iron us out too. By upsetting the balance of nature by artificially reducing the birth rate we are frustrating the innate natural rhythms of life and causing a back lash. The visible backlash at present is the actual disappearance of the races and gene pools that are contracepting. In another 25 years the European gene pool will be in danger of serious decline. As it stands most countries are not reproducing their population. The numbers of immigrants is increasing in these countries and this trend is rising and shows no sign of stopping. These are facts. The real demographic problem is under population in the developed countries. The real other problem is that these very countries are actively exporting this malady to Africa, India China etc. Given this trend in 50 years swathes of the planet will be old and infirm and the young population will have dwindled to single figures. This is the backlash of a worldwide contraceptive practice. When you look at the maths and forecast graphs you see that this contraceptive trend is chronic, contagious and decimates races and peoples. Absence of widespread contraception allows each continent or country to thrive and be autonomous and nature's ebbs and flows continue and man's numbers will not suffocate the planet but the bad behaviour of a few could.

The CIA website on world facts shows in graph form the reproductive figures for 224 countries. The vast majority score less than 2.1 children per woman, the vital number needed to replace the population, which means these countries have a declining population. They are not reproducing themselves and are eventually heading for dwindling numbers unless the trend is stopped. These are stark facts and rocketing health budgets in the Western world confirm the trend of the aging population with multiple health needs.

THE TIP OF THE ICEBERG

Iran has had a population growth in the past 75 years and now numbers 75 million, more than half of whom are under 35 years of age. They are projected to reach 100 million by 2050. A scientific Iranian journal article reports that the level of breast cancer incidence there is 17.1 per 100,000 person years whereas it is 99.4 for USA and 83 for Western Europe and 46 for Eastern Europe. The figures for other Asian countries using the same methods are 25 to 30. These are really big differences. They explain away these differences in the article by attributing them to environmental exposures, lifestyle differences, and also to the presence of screening in affluent countries causing early detection of invasive cancers. (A. Sadjadi et al. La Revue de Sante de la Mediteranee orientale. Vol 15, No.6. 2009).

This article also shows that in the most deprived area where women had many children and breast fed and did not use OCs the breast cancer rate was the lowest. This is the province of Ardabil. They further explain why the breast cancer rates are so low. This is not a major publication in the breast cancer world and those that do not like the findings can easily attribute them to poor design, lack of appropriate controls and ill defined diagnostic techniques. They then can and do minimize the results by saying they are due to environment, life style, and reproductive patterns. The truth of this small study from Iran, and there are many from all over Asia and Pakistan and India also, is that the facts are there for all to see. The incidence of breast cancer in these countries is 80% less than it is in USA and Western Europe. That is an incontrovertible fact. That is gross and amazing and what is sure is that the answer to the breast cancer epidemic in the West is contained in this simple study from Iran. Why are the figures so largely different? The answer is that they were not exposed to the same level of female hormone hit that the Western world is exposed to on a daily basis due to OCs and HRT.

They reference an interesting paper in their own discussion piece from 2005 from Dumitrescu RG in The Journal of Cellular and Molecular Medicine, where it catalogues the causes of breast cancer. Looking at this table it looks like a level playing field with no "one" factor towering over the others. This cannot be true since Iran and Asia has up to 80% less breast cancer than USA. There must be a towering cause to give this result. This is the same problem that has dogged breast cancer research for decades. Good simple and raw data is taken and stood on its head and scientists and doctors argue over what could be the correct conclusion and meantime the real elephant of greatly increased breast cancer incidence is ignored. This is a classic case of what has been going on and why breast cancer is still the scourge it is in the West. The satellite picture shows breast cancer hot spots in USA, Western Europe, Japan and very little in Asia, Africa, Pakistan. An identikit picture shows the usage of HRT and OCs exactly the same colours over these areas.

The website of Earth Policy Institute shows that Europe and USA have usage of OCs of 36 and 24 couples per 100 whereas in Asia it is 10. The breast cancer incidence is a mirror image of this. The big news story stands out and no matter what amount of explaining away it is still a fact and true, and unless honesty prevails and the facts are accepted the breast cancer problem will never be sorted.

This is a further aspect of the entire debacle. How the really important and simple truth is ignored and obfuscated. This is simple data. Take 100 women on the pill for 10 years and 100 women not on it and over 35 or 50 years compare the incidence of breast cancer. Take a country where it is common and one where it is uncommon and look to see why they differ. Treat 100s of lab mammals with feed containing contraceptives and another few 100 with contraceptive free feed and over time compare the incidence of breast cancer. The studies are easy but the results to date of millions of women studied are confusing. There is something unusual about that. There must be a reason why simple comparative studies such as these have been so confusing and contradictory for decades now. It is the first time in 100 years that a cause for an illness has taken so long to find with so many people involved in it and so much money spent on it. The big data satellite picture shows the reality and maybe that is where the answer is.

The World Breast Cancer Report 2012 (published by The International Prevention Research Institute) and presented at The National Cancer Institute Directors Meeting USA reports a 3.1% annual increase in breast cancer worldwide over the past 30 years. In 1980 there were 640,000 cases compared to 1.6 million in 2012. They call it a call to arms against breast cancer and a real cancer pandemic. These words are based on facts and are delivered by serious people with genuine concern for the ongoing and escalating scourge of breast cancer. A look at an underdeveloped country like Pakistan (Journal of Pakistan Medical Association. Gilani G.M. Oct 2003) and reading an article about breast cancer there shows three things. (1) The incidence and death from breast cancer in Pakistan is about 60% lower than in the western world. (2) They look with dismay at the large numbers in the Western world with breast cancer. Breast cancer is the most common cancer in women in Pakistan but only 1 to 2 % of women there are treated for breast cancer on reaching their 65th birthday. This is very different to the west where the incidence is 1 in 10 women. This significant and cannot be diluted and ignored by putting it down to climate or food or late presentation. (3) Women in less developed countries present later in the course of breast cancer and do not do as well because they present too late in the course of the illness. The mortality from breast cancer is similar in developed countries to underdeveloped countries because they have better and earlier treatments in developed countries and obviously bigger numbers of cases in developed countries (Breast cancer report).

Perusal of The Surgeon General's annual 2013 National Prevention Strategy makes no mention of breast cancer. Walking and tobacco are priorities and other good interventions but no campaign to eradicate cancer inducing female hormones such as OCs or HRT. This shows the mind set of the leaders and although everything in the report you may or may not agree with breast cancer should be there. These initiatives also mean money toward preferred projects, and the absolute cost in suffering, deaths and finance caused by breast cancer is enormous, and would easily repay any money spent on an advertisement campaign warning women of the risks of hormones (OCs, HRT) in causing breast cancer. The National Cancer Institute USA says that there will be 232,000 new cases of breast cancer in USA in 2013 and 39,000 deaths from it. It goes on to say in the official SEER database that between 2006 and 2010, 1.8% of women who got breast cancer were between 20 and 34 years old, 9.6% were between ages 35 and 44, 22.2% were between 45 and 54 years old. This equates by simple maths to 33.6% who got breast cancer in those years were 54 years old or younger. This calculates at 77,952 cases per year or a total of 389,760 for the 5 years. These are staggering figures for young women and require drastic action.

With this in mind you go to the search engine on the site and input "breast cancer and the oral contraceptive" and you get a sheet telling you among other things; "OCs increase the incidence of breast cancer slightly in current users and particularly in young women. This risk returns to normal levels after 10 years being off the OC. OCs also reduce the incidence of ovarian and endometrial cancer and the protective effect is greater the longer the OCs are taken." This is definitely not a "Government health Warning not to take OCs or HRT for fear of breast cancer statement" one would have expected seeing the enormous numbers of young women contracting the disease in USA. This is a very weak warning statement from an official organ of cancer research and advocacy. This statement is typical of all the official sites that cover breast cancer. Write to any of the official cancer centres or medical journals and the same "slight risk" statements emerge.

MORE STRAWS IN THE WIND

Big simple pictures don't lie. When you look up and there is a big black cloud overhead and at the same time on the radio you hear the weatherman telling you it is a sunny day, who do you think is right? Weather men and women do get it right a good deal of the time but also get it terribly wrong. Your own eyes and experience are correct and the weather man is wrong "for you" whatever about the rest of the country. When patterns show that the lower a population's fertility is the greater the breast cancer incidence is, you conclude that there seems to be a connection between having babies and breast cancer. The less babies the more breast cancer. This pattern is well recognised and even if it wasn't all you have to do is make your own graph. Put births in a country on one side and numbers with breast cancer on another, and you see immediately that the lower the birth rate the higher the breast cancer numbers. This is simple it is the black cloud and the weather man has gotten it wrong.

This was shown more scientifically in a research article in the Demographic Research Journal in 15 April 2008 called "Cohort fertility patterns and breast mortality among US women, 1948-2003," by Krueger et al. They showed that in US the deaths from breast cancer corresponded to the decline in births at a certain young age. This is a well trodden path in all developed countries and asks the question what has low birth rate got to do with breast cancer? The other way to look at this issue is to ask how a population lowers it's birth rate significantly from on average 4 or 5 children per family to 1or 2? The answer to this may help to point to a cause of the breast cancer. For example: (1) Does having few or no babies itself increase breast cancer risk? There is reliable evidence that shows the more children a woman has the significantly less breast cancer she gets. Some put this figure as high as 50% less chance of breast cancer for having 4 or 5 children compared to having none. This is even better if the first child was had before 20 years of age. The younger the first baby the better the reduction in breast cancer risk. The reason is thought to be the reduction of exposure to ovarian sex hormones from menstrual cycle reduction by multiple pregnancies and also breast feeding. The evidence is less clear on whether the very fact of not having children itself is carcinogenic but more likely the means used to be infertile (OCs) may be the underlying cause of increase in breast cancer risk. (2) Having said this the epidemiology of fertility and its control leading to a population reduction in birth rate, indicates some new factor in the population causing widespread infertility. Enter the oral contraceptives. Their growth in use is mirrored by a similar reduction in birth rate and a simultaneous increase in breast cancer incidence.

These three graphs of entire populations across the world are too consistent and robust to be mere chance or insignificant. They actually are the raw data underlying the present and spreading increase of breast cancer. Countries that use more OCs and other means of birth control and have fewer children as a consequence have more breast cancer per woman. This increase in breast cancer is mainly in the oestrogen receptor sensitive type, the type that extra oestrogen (OCs) would ignite. The breast cancer data on lifetime exposure to oestrogen is very strong. The more menstrual cycles and therefore oestrogen exposure a woman has in her lifetime the higher the risk of getting breast cancer. Any thing that reduces the overall exposure to oestrogen over a lifetime reduces the risk e.g. multiple pregnancies carried to term, breast feeding, ophorectomy (removal of ovaries which are the source of female sex hormones).

It seems very clear that if you give more oestrogen and progestin this will not reduce the risk but actually increase it. This is because of the increased oestrogen load a woman is exposed to and as we have seen from previous data, more oestrogen means more cancer. What is also emerging is that early exposure to oestrogen causes increased risk of breast cancer for example with early menarche or OCs taken in the teens and thereafter.

The National Cancer Institute US makes several points under the heading

"Reproductive history and breast cancer risk":

- The hormonal changes that occur during pregnancy may influence a woman's chance of developing breast cancer later in life.
- Some factors associated with pregnancy may reduce a woman's chance of developing breast cancer later in life.
- Some factors associated with pregnancy may increase a woman's chance of developing breast cancer.
- Induced abortion and miscarriage have not been shown to increase a woman's chance of developing breast cancer.
- Pregnancy may reduce a woman's chance of developing some other cancers, including ovarian, and endometrial cancers, later in life.

These points are further expanded on and say that a woman's risk of breast cancer is related to her exposure to hormones that are produced by her ovaries (endogenous oestrogen and progesterone). Reproductive factors that increase the duration and/or levels of exposure to ovarian hormones, which stimulate cell growth, have been associated with an increase in breast cancer risk. These factors include early onset of menstruation, late onset of menopause, later age at first pregnancy, and never having given birth. They do not comment on why a woman never gave birth. For example was it a lifestyle choice or because she was infertile or because she had an illness or because she was using birth control? These confounders have an obvious impact on the suggested relationship between never giving birth and increased risk of breast cancer.

They say that pregnancy and breast feeding both reduce a woman's lifetime number of menstrual cycles, and thus her cumulative exposure to endogenous (oestrogen and progesterone) hormones. In addition they add that pregnancy and breast feeding have a direct effect on breast cells, causing them to differentiate or mature so that they can produce milk. Some say theses cells resist cancer better than ones that do not differentiate (see references to article). Thus they conclude that (1) early age at first pregnancy (2) increasing number of births (3) history of preeclampsia and (4) longer duration of breast feeding all decrease risk of breast cancer. The jury is out on abortion because of complicating factors, but it definitely does not reduce the risk and many authors say it increases the risk.

Dr Chris Kahlenborn has sifted through the publications on breast cancer and the pill in his book published in 2000 called "Breast Cancer: its link to abortion and the birth control pill," available on Amazon.com. He reports a significantly increased risk of breast cancer with OC use. His interview in May 2000 with the Federal Drugs Administration published on the web is very revealing and concise regarding the evidence for and against the pill—breast cancer connection, and in their final roundup they ask the following question:

"Can you give an overall statement regarding early OC use and breast cancer" to which he replies:

"If a woman takes the oral contraceptive pill before her first child is born, she suffers a 40% increase risk of developing breast cancer compared to women who do not take the pill. If she takes OCs for 4 years or more prior to her first baby, she suffers at least a 72% increased risk for developing breast cancer."

These are very big numbers but no bigger than you would have expected given the population numbers with breast cancer and the recent data showing aggressive breast cancer in younger women. Other even more alarming figures are quoted in his testimony including a 210% increased risk in young women who took OCs for 10 or more years having begun to take them before age 18 years. This FDA interview and his book are among the more comprehensive documents testifying to the risk of breast cancer with OCs. These data and his testimony before the FDA are unrefuted and uncontested it seems. He lists many of the research papers pointing out the risks of breast cancer from OCs and they are readily available to anyone who wants to see them in his book.

Lynn Rosenberg in the American Journal of Epidemiology 2009; 169, also found the same significant increase in risk with OCs. Samuel Epstein of University of Illinois at Chicago has fairly strong words for the companies producing the new "low dose" mini pills when he points out that the low dose synthetic ethinyl estradiol is 40 times more potent than the natural estradiol thus constituting a much bigger hormonal hit. (Cancer Prevention Coalition). These researchers among hundreds of others trade data, graphs and risk figures which seem trustworthy, credible, and consistent with opposing data from the other camp who write in the top journals—The Lancet, New England journal of Medicine and British medical journal, contradicting their figures and saying there is no or little risk.

This is the landscape and the reason why this issue will never be resolved by experts is simply because it is tit for tat behaviour which will never reach a conclusion. A new approach is needed to expose the truth of the issue. Ignore the experts and see what you think yourself. Look at the crude and original data the actual numbers with breast cancer, their ages, what countries have more than others and then think . . . . why?

Looking at today's web edition of The British Medical Journal three major articles jump out.

(1) Different combined oral contraceptives and the risk of venous thrombosis: a systematic review and network meta-analysis by Stegeman et al 12.9.2013. This looked for a primary outcome of fatal or non fatal first episode venous thrombosis (blood clot) or pulmonary embolism (clot in the lung) in those taking OCs. The age profile was of young women of reproductive age and they found an average increase of risk of three and a half times compared to those not on OCs and this risk rising to six fold for certain pill types.

(2) Quantification of harms in cancer screening trials: literature review by Heleno et al. 5.10.2013. This was a comprehensive trawl through good quality publications on cancer screening to see if they reported side effects of the actual screening process itself and its sequelae. They found that the most important harms of screening (over diagnosis and false positive findings) were only reported in 7% and 4% of studies. They also reference data which is based on systematic reviews of cancer screening trials, that say that screening has either modest or no effect in reducing cancer mortality.

(3) "Hardly worth the effort"? Medical journals' policies and their editors' and publishers' views on trial registration and publication bias: quantitative and qualitative study. By Wager et al 6.9.2013. This looked at trial registration which reduces publication bias. From 200 journals they studied only 55 required trial registration and 3 actively discouraged it. They suggested that competition between journals was a factor in why there was such a low uptake in trial registration.

These three articles highlight the minefield that published research is and the daunting and often impossible task it is to separating genuine data from spurious statistics and spin. The article about thrombosis and OCs is alerting in the fact that these risk numbers are high and constitute a serious side effect in young women. The screening article is of note because it shows a widespread lack of full disclosure or evaluation of serious harms, and also states that screening is not a proven effective intervention for reducing mortality in any cancer management. The publication article shows a patchy standard in medical journal articles and a bias factor in a real and tangible example. The implication is that if bias is abundant in this small area it must also be occurring in a widespread fashion in medical publication. A downstream effect of this is poor decision making. Policy and treatments and interventions are based on such literature, and incorrect protocols and interventions are approved because of a less than perfect evidence base, with resulting poor or even worse results for patients. These deviations are all relevant to the published literature on breast cancer and have all contributed to muddying the waters. The proof is that we are still no where near arresting its advance.

So the first clear and undisputed fact is that breast cancer is getting much more common and now approaches 1.6 million cases this year alone compared to 0.6 million 30 years ago. This is confirmed by all the major cancer institutes and international databases and also by a major review article in The Lancet 2011 entitled: "Breast and Cervical Cancer in 187 countries between 1980 and 2010; a systematic analysis." The SEER database and the UK Cancer Institute show that the numbers of young women of less than 54 years down to late teens with breast cancer is very high and these younger women also have the worst aggressive type of cancer. (Reference and figures given previously). The bulk of breast cancer is in developed countries with remote countries having up to 80% less incidence of breast cancer. These developed countries do not have a similar spike in cancer of any other species nor is there a similar peak and increase in cancer in young males. Thus it is just the relatively young females that are singled out. The incidence of cancers in similarly aged young males is actually half of the numbers it is in females. The unnatural pattern of a cancer affecting young women in a very aggressive way is notable. It is unique in occurrence since no other mammal has such a peak and nor do men.

The question has to be: what are young women in developed countries doing or what are they exposed to that men and animals in those same countries are not exposed to or doing, and to which young women in underdeveloped countries are not exposed to or doing either? The answer to that question is the pointer to the cause of the breast cancer epidemic.

MORE EVIDENCE

More recent data published on the incidence of breast cancer in young women comes from USA. (Journal of the Medical Association of America Feb 27th 2013). It again is bad news and shows that there was a statistically significant increase in the incidence of breast cancer with secondary spread, in USA between 1976 and 2009 for women aged 25 to 39 years without a corresponding increase in older women. In fact the figures nearly doubled from 1.53 per 100,000 to 2.9 per 100,000 young women in this time frame. This was a comprehensive article based on the SEER database and carried in one of the most important American journals.

It further goes on to confirm that the 25 to 39 year age group have the lowest 5 year survival rate for this type of breast cancer. (Approximately 30% are alive after 5 years). Similar trends were reported in Switzerland and they also cannot identify a likely cause for the continued and worsening incidence of this more aggressive breast cancer type in this young age group. A particular finding was that the increase in aggressive breast cancer was significantly more common in "oestrogen positive receptor type breast cancer" which is certainly consistent with an increased oestrogen load (from OCs) causing an increased cancer incidence. This they do not say but advance the usual suspects of lifestyle, diet, obesity etc. But why not state the obvious? The article gives 14 references from reputable journals again reporting increased aggressive breast cancer in young women over the recent years.

The lead author also reports that the incidence of advanced breast cancer in young women has been increasing by 2% annually since the 1970s and shows no sign of abating. In The Los Angeles Times the study authors suggest that the cause of the increase in aggressive breast cancer in young women is due to lifestyle changes that occurred during the study period. Diet, exercise, obesity, earlier on set menstruation, use of birth control, delayed pregnancy and other factors may play a role. They do not advise any particular preventative measures except to advise that yes serious breast cancer can and does occur in young women and it is on the increase. In another similar interview with The New York Times Dr Johnson the lead author repeated the facts. This time dissenting voices were appended in the form of educated commentary from experts and most of these played down the findings. The advocacy group for young women with breast cancer, Young Survival Coalition, through their spokeswoman Michelle Esser said they were looking with caution at the data and said that improved diagnostic or staging tests might account for the apparent increase. "We don't want to invite panic or alarm".

This then is a classical case of serious data published in a prestigious journal being assessed and reported and possibly shelved, from the point of view of highlighting the major issue of causation of this surge in serious breast cancer. The brightest and best in newspaper reporters and medical oncologists talk readily about the show and the cast and the background music but make scant reference to the producer.

That is the question. What or who is behind the constant increase in breast cancer numbers and why is it happening at all? They all agree it is scary and awful and . . . . "Is it true what this article is saying? The results need to be replicated in other countries and really it is too early to comment," which of course is correct but . . . . the cause, the producer of this tragedy who or what is causing it is ignored. They sidestep the biggest gouger in the room.

It sounds like "déjà vu all over again!" This is the pattern of breast cancer research reporting to date and it shows how it causes and does not halt the advance and escalation of the terrible spread of this illness. The brightest and the best lock horns about the minutiae of the issue and meanwhile the war rages on and the camouflaged enemy is again behind the advancing line (OCs, HRT). This type of behaviour characterises the insidious pattern of negating good data by directing the focus away from a key finding causing it to be forgotten about, and then focussing attention on less important issues and thus neutralizing it's impact. This allows the breast cancer pandemic to progress with the result of millions of breast cancer deaths and untold grief to young unsuspecting women and their friends and families. Turning a blind eye to the real causation of a serious ongoing (50 years) epidemic that picks out young women is serious particularly since it could have been stopped decades ago. It is now gathering momentum and attacking the third world, with the knowledge and foresight of those who should be trying to stop it.

What will happen now is that other countries and data bases of aggressive breast cancer in young women will publish their findings and a clear picture is unlikely to emerge for 3 reasons.

(1) Their findings will not agree; in which case doubt is cast on the veracity of the SEER data and it is sidelined.

(2) The findings agree and a significant increase in aggressive breast cancer in young women world wide (developed world) is confirmed, but then all the experts will focus on early detection, or new treatments or screening or other aspects of the problem and completely ignore the causation issue. This has occurred since the beginning of this breast cancer epidemic and unfortunately will continue to happen unless patient advocacy groups and journalists speak up. No one will point at the cause with courage and single mindedness and say "it's the pill".

(3) The findings in the US will be a stand out and the figures from other countries (with maybe less credible data bases) will be mixed in with those from the US in a metanalysis and the definitive findings from this super metanalysis will show no or minimal increase in aggressive breast cancer in young women. This will then be taken as the gold standard and watershed

statement and adopted by all the associations and medical bodies as the last word . . . . and we are back on our heads again. The aetiology of breast cancer will be delayed by another 35 years. This is what we are living through now because the gold standard, watershed metanalyses of the 80s and 90s are still accepted as the last word and anyone who suggests anything else is ignored and ostracized.

Among these stand out The Lancet paper of 1996, and The Million women study (which showed that HRT greatly increased breast cancer), and the 2002 Marchbanks study in the New England Journal of Medicine which all reassured women and doctors that there is no real risk with OCs and breast cancer incidence. These and similar studies and metanalyses have succeeded in turning the collective gaze of scientists and doctors away from hormones (OCs and HRT) as a cause of breast cancer.

Let us peruse the web site of Susan G. Komen a great name in breast cancer struggle and one of the very first sites that you see on googling "breast cancer and oral contraceptives". What you would expect from such a site would be a woman friendly and truthful steer on OCs. It says that:

"Present or recent use of birth control pills slightly increases risk of breast cancer".

The blurb on HRT is ambivalent:

"Longer term use of oestrogen plus progestin increases breast cancer risk. The risk declines over time once a woman stops taking hormones. Findings on menopausal hormone use (with oestrogen alone) are mixed. Some show these hormones increase breast cancer risk and others do not . . . . ask your doctor about risks and benefits." Further on when it poses the question: "The risk of breast cancer for women who are currently taking birth control pills?" The answer is:

"Studies have shown current or recent use of birth control pills slightly increase breast cancer risk. Most of these studies were done on older forms of the pill. There is not enough research to know whether or not "mini-pills" affect breast cancer risk the same as other types of birth control pills".

Next: "Women who have stopped using birth control pills should they be concerned about their risk of breast cancer?" Answer:

"Once stopped, the risk decreases over time. After about 10 years of not using birth control pills a woman's risk is the same as a woman who never took the pills". This is added to in another section where it says to young women: "Although taking the pill slightly increases the risk, most women on the pill are at low risk of breast cancer because they are young and premenopausal. So even with a slight increase in risk they are still unlikely to get breast cancer. And once women stop taking the pill the slight increase in risk begins to decrease and over time goes away".

The take home message is anything but "stop the pill". It is reassuring in tone in saying that yes there is slight risk but it disappears when you stop. Mini-pills and newer HRT are rehabilitated by saying that there is not enough research done to say one way or the other if they pose a risk. This is a site for lay people not doctors only and so it's body language says "don't worry" and the impact statement's subliminal message is like "it's ok to take the pill but do be careful". This is again tacit endorsement for birth control pills without showing the raw incidence data for breast cancer and very likely connection between OCs and breast cancer. This is a breast cancer awareness or support and information site supposedly for the wellbeing of women but it actually does the opposite to what it should do. It should warn women forcefully of the continual increase in breast cancer incidence, of the rising numbers of young women with aggressive and often fatal breast cancer, and of the obvious connection between oestrogen receptor positive breast cancer and exposure to female hormones.

The Million Women Study from Oxford UK was a wake up call for the HRT industry and menopausal and post menopausal women. It was and is a study of over one million women aged 50 years or more led by Dame Valerie Beral. It along with the Women's Health Initiative study in USA confirmed a very significant increase in breast cancer in women taking HRT. The use of HRT in many countries dropped by figures of more than 50% following this publication and cancer of the breast also decrease in tandem. This then was a successful and thorough study whose findings did live to see the light of day and impacted on policy statements from the Royal College of Obstetricians and Gynaecologists and from The Commission on Human Medicines who changed their recommendations on prescribing and use of HRT. You may well ask what the difference is between this effect of HRT on breast cancer incidence and that of OCs and the answer is not much if any. Both cause increased female hormone loads on females in one case premenopausal and in the other postmenopausal, and both are known to increase breast cancer incidence.

The optics for OCs however are different for 3 reasons.

(1) The obvious one is the "Slight risk story or slogan" which successfully detoxes the risk element for women and encourages them not to change their OC behaviour "but to be careful".
(2) The second is the reproductive repercussions and what it means to the social psyche to realise that the pill which was promoted as the cure all for women, is not that in fact but on the contrary a very significant cause of breast cancer in women. This is a hard "pill" to swallow and

is absolutely counter cultural and flies in the face of all the advice women have been reading in magazines and websites and in official pronouncements on the pill.

(3) Lastly the drugs market for OCs is enormous and has a very big interest in protecting its products. Could it be the cigarette controversy all over again?

COLLECTIVE MYOPIA

A similar professional myopia and blindness occurred recently in UK with the Mid Staffordshire hospital disaster. It was not the doctors or nurses or administration that spoke up about the awful care and rocketing death count in the hospital but patient advocates and a local journalist. This then spawned into the 1700 page Francis report which pulled the wool from the eyes of all and showed the terrible conditions in the hospital and made 290 recommendations. This had big downstream effects in that other hospitals were investigated and the Liverpool Care Pathway was decommissioned and stopped. This was a fully accredited end of life "care pathway" used all over UK and was instrumental in many untimely deaths at Mid Staffordshire. This should never have gotten that far. Those in charge should have seen the problems but they were distracted by other issues. In this case it was the budget and cost cutting in their attempt to achieve trust status. The result was that they took their eyes of the ball and the whole enterprise came tumbling down. This is a common occurrence in any corporate failure. It happens when the—"back to basics and why we are here and what are the key things we should be doing," leaflet which is the mission statement of the outfit, is put safely in a drawer and forgotten about, and attention is focussed on secondary and lesser targets and then not surprisingly disaster strikes.

THE MEDICS AND SCIENTISTS WILL NOT SOLVE THE BREAST CANCER ISSUE.

Try writing to a medical journal or paper and saying that you think the OCs and HRT are causing the breast cancer epidemic. You may get a polite thank you and silence. It will be the patient power and a savvy small-time journalist or local radio show that will blow the whole thing into orbit. Then there will be awesome backtracking and blame flinging and serious galloping to the trenches for cover. This has to happen because this disaster cannot be allowed to continue.

OK let's take another route. What if you had a vested interest and wanted the OCs and HRT to not only continue to sell and spread but wanted seriously to expand the market? What would you do how and take us through it. A similar ploy is used with the alcohol or gun lobby and look at their success. Despite repetitive mass shootings and shopping mall carnage the gun lobby has held firm and even quick high volume magazine weapons continue to be readily available. The alcoholics business is burgeoning and in some places like UK beer is cheaper than water. The governments of US and UK are hamstrung by the drinks industry and have even joined with the abstinence groups to help people to "drink sensibly". How smart is that! To promote OCs and HRT you do a number of things:

1.   You get real time data on how the drugs are selling, where they are selling and what the profits are.

2. You extrapolate to see how to sustain and grow the business.
3. You search for big new markets and go after them.
4. You see the obstacles and what could stop your plan.
5. You develop an effective strategy to neutralise opposition or obstacles.

Number 5 is the interesting one. How do you do this? You strengthen the marketing and advertisement and edge over opposition by having better advertisements, cheaper goods, or cleaner side effect profiles. To counteract any damage from side effect data coming out you neutralise it or if possible block it coming out. So you pay off big hitters (prestigious medics or scientists) and they do the business by suppressing unwanted publicity or disclosure of nasty side effects. You fund your own "rigorous studies" overtly or covertly with the really big names that will hold clout and tell them what results you would really like to see. You then get these papers published in top medical journals having first trouble shot them with statistical wizards and software packages that could make digital reimaging look like an archived cave find. You buy web sites promoting breast cancer treatment and tips and champion Pink Ribbon initiatives. You have then successfully hijacked the cause and everyone looks to you for direction. The wolf in sheep's clothing syndrome.

To really scupper the ideological opposition you join them and if possible get a leadership or committee role. Then there is no one as zealous as you and your team in finding initiatives and support groups and fundraising events, to really get a handle on the breast cancer scourge that is killing all these young people. You make statements carried by the wires, you go to Congress looking for research funding . . . . and meantime like the Pied Piper you draw all in sundry in a merry dance behind your altruistic campaign and successfully take the spotlight off your product the pill. Job done. Then you keep abreast of developments and threats to business and deploy experts to quench any dissenting voices (like neutralising the JAMA paper above) and carry on. To really embed your mission statement in structures you get it accepted as dogma by getting a really big person to endorse it. Enter Melinda Gates and the Millennium Goals and the "unmet contraceptive needs of the third world". This is the new lingo and all the wise caps tout it and all the big journals flaunt it and third world countries are buying into it because they are (1) fooled, (2) won't get money unless they give out the pills, (3) they possibly haven't had time to analyse the raw data and see the devastating effects of OC policy in the West.

This is a very successful, or disastrous more correctly said, obstacle to getting to the truth of the problem. Why? Because for whatever reason these key studies (Lancet, Marchbanks etc) have closed off any serious consideration that the real culprit of breast cancer could actually be the most obvious (OCs, HRT) and have succeeded in directing the focus onto other things like: treatment, receptor type, relative differences from country to country or genetics of cancer etc. These are important areas but should not usurp the primary area of concern which is that of causation and subsequent prevention. Why are these studies (the Lancet, Marchbanks and others) wrong? They are wrong for 5 reasons:

1. The breast cancer statistics world wide contradict them by continuing to report increases and worsening in numbers and severity (deaths in young women especially from aggressive breast cancer). That is the raw data and it continues to show that there is a very real breast cancer cause that has not been targeted. The risk they (Lancet, Marchbanks etc) attribute to OCs has to be seriously underestimated.

2. They have successfully eliminated any root and branch investigation into OCs in the causation of breast cancer by having big names big numbers and big journals backing their results. Who can compete with that show of strength? This has allowed the epidemic to continue and grow.

3. They were not independent government sponsored studies but mainly metanalyses which though useful are not gold standard randomly controlled trials free from vested interest and bias.

4. They did not convincingly and transparently show they were drug company free and unbiased.

5. The background noise is all wrong. There is definite data to prove the unremitting progress of the ravages of breast cancer. (Recent data cited in this article). The topic of OCs is a fully blown example of a potentially bias laden subject. The odds are absolutely against an unbiased result for this issue because there is too much money, too much ideology, and too much desire for the pill to be endorsed as safe and well for any other result to be palatable or acceptable. The proof is to look at the myriads of breast cancer publications that contradict one another and the absence of a clear consensus after all the research and conferences and meetings . . . . sponsored by OH Yes! . . . . The drugs industry!

Spin and bias is enormous in published studies of breast cancer trials. This was highlighted in the January 2013 edition of the prestigious journal Annals of Oncology in the article: "Bias in reporting of end points of efficacy and toxicity in randomized clinical trials for women with breast cancer", where the lead researcher of the paper Ian Tannock states that they found bias in adverse effect reporting in 2 thirds of papers reviewed with poor reporting also of more serious side effects. One third of trials were reported as positive even though their primary out come target did not show a significant benefit.

This is the calibre of high impact articles in really good journals and displays a very dodgy evidence base. This is in the world of treatments for breast cancer and the dollars are at stake, so fudging data and spinning results means more possible sales and more money as a result. This is no different to any branch of medicine or any endeavour where the stakes are high and the pressures to succeed are great and the competition with rivals is fierce. The influence of bias infects everyone's integrity unless rigorous safeguards are in place and are marshalled by independent and even "blind" assessors. The contagion effect also kicks in as; "well if they're all at it we can't get left behind or we will go under" type of situation. Just look at the two commonest topics some journalists report at the Olympic athlete's quarters: "Who is making how much money? Who is taking what drug?" It sounds terrible but what about Lance Armstrong and his 7 consecutive Tour de France medals? The pundits suspected something and it took a seriously energized journalist to find the truth. The Watergate scandal was also a major outage by what some would call a courageous article in Washington Post of 9 August 1974 by journalists Woodward and Bernstein.

These and many more untouchables and unthinkables have gone belly up in the spotlight and it all started with straws in the wind and inklings and suspicions that all was not as it is seemed to be. Breast cancer is a much thornier issue from a possible cover up or camouflage or bias point of view. The reason is because it is embedded in the scientific and medical culture that breast cancer is not caused to any significant degree by the pill. This is accepted dogma. This is the 7-Tour de France medal statement "I am clean", this is the athlete's mess room clamour "we don't do drugs", this is The Presidents defence of innocence, and yet he barely escaped being the first president indicted for felonies committed in of all places the Oval Office.

The other pressures brought to bear on breast cancer are the drug industry interest and their finances and the ideological birth control lobby with its vested interests. Among the key players in any war or competition rank the media. To win the war and lose the media war is defeat in many people's books. Propaganda is a powerful agent for change and lobbying is a well respected element of any political or social establishment. Thus all the ducks have to be in a row to win. To be right and not be seen to be right is next to useless as regards social traction or power to change people's attitude and behaviour. So the war is waged simultaneously on many fronts and each of them has to be in synchrony.

The press coverage of the pill and breast cancer has been like a summer of forest fires. Breaking news about a possible risk of breast cancer from the pill gets bold headlines only to be rubbished in the next edition by some expert saying the opposite and watering things down. There is relative calm in the media at present about breast cancer and they are content to publish human interest stories of cures or deaths or possible breakthroughs in treatment. They do not neglect the topic and how could they with 232,000 new cases of invasive breast cancer per year in USA and 40,000 deaths.

Doing simple maths that would be 2.3 million new cases in 10 years and 4.6 million in 20 years on top of the other sufferers. In total 12% of American women will get breast cancer according to the official cancer USA site. There were 156 million women in USA in 2009 and 12% is 18.7 million which is an awful lot of women affected by the disease not to mention those investigated or biopsied or treated or just worried. This is a major health issue and the media watch it carefully. The media are fed the official public health speak of "slight risk". This of course is great official speak and who would deny a woman her just rights? But why not tell the whole truth? Why not add a warning that "you could get clots, a stroke, breast cancer, weight gain, bloating . . ." and "to tell the truth at least 19 million women in USA have breast cancer as we speak and to be honest some say the pill is a real big cause" . . . . also "the fertility number in USA at present is 1.88 children per woman which is not even replacing the population" (the figure needed is 2.1). These parts of complete disclosure are omitted.

Shakespeare put similar inklings in the mouth of Marcellus in the play Hamlet when he said: "Something is rotten in the state of Denmark". Hamlet meets Horatio on the battlements of the castle just before midnight. In the darkness they hear raucous laughter and dancing. The King gulps his "draughts of Rhenish down" and all around is debauchery. Marcellus utters this line in sighs of woe at the festering moral and political corruption. Horatio retorts: "Heaven will direct it" meaning that heaven will protect Denmark. Francisco a minor character agrees with Marcellus and says: "For this relief much thanks; 'tis bitter cold and I am sick at heart". This play was one of Shakespeare's great tragedies and these quotes capture the foreboding and gathering storm clouds over the state. A similar foreboding can be sensed around the coverage and denial of a real problem with the state of breast cancer.

It is a Donald Rumsfeld moment. The now famous statement of the 21st United States Secretary of Defence highlighted the "unknown unknowns". Quoted in full he said "Reports that say that something hasn't happened are always interesting to me, because as we know, there are known knowns; these are things we know we know. We also know there are known unknowns; that is to say we know there are some things we do not know. But there are also unknown unknowns—the ones we don't know we don't know. And if one looks throughout the history of our country and other free countries, it is the latter category that tend to be the difficult ones." "The absence of evidence is not evidence of absence, or vice versa."

A similar annunciation could be invoked to capture the breast cancer world. There are many knowns. Look at any website and click on risk factors for breast cancer. A cascade of low medium and high risk items appear. There are some notables like a strong family history, or previous breast cancer or strong genetic loading but after that it is amorphous and featureless. There is no red flag. The prognosis for various types and stages of the cancer are knowns. The response rates to various treatments are knowns. The countries that have most and least breast cancer are knowns. The rise and rise and rise of its incidence is known. The high risk of HRT for breast cancer is a known. The known unknowns are: Why did it all start? What will be the situation in another decade? How come poorer countries don't get it next to nearly as much as USA or Western Europe? Why don't young men and animals get some similar form of cancer? These lists are not exhaustive.

The really interesting ones as Rumsfeld states are the unknown unknowns. What could there be out there that we haven't even thought of? A terrorist group infecting the developed world water supply with carcinogens? No? Avian flu morphing into airborne carcinogenic particles targeting females only? No? Cosmetics with heretofore unrecognised carcinogenic properties? No? Maybe it is a mirage and someone is cooking the books and it really isn't happening? No? Maybe loads of important people know the unknown unknowns? Yes?

The unknown unknowns for the average woman and doctor and drug representative are not unknown unknowns to everyone. Someone knows. The absence of evidence is not evidence of the absence of this truth. Let's stand back and look at the big picture. There are several major players in this tragedy. The leading lady is unfortunately the young woman with aggressive breast cancer. The second lady is the middle aged or more elderly woman with breast cancer. The main actor is a ghost. He is not seen or heard and yet is all over the place directing the entire drama. He is multifaceted and has many costumes. He owns big drug companies, he fronts breast cancer support sites, he organises breast cancer information days and conferences and has a spin off in breast cancer merchandise like hand bags and sweat shirts and sportswear. He bankrolls media campaigns and is ahead of the curve with what is fresh and breaking news in the research and medical journal world. He seeks new markets for low-low dose mini-mini pills and lobbies Congress to "for God's sake help the poor in those countries to have safe maternal health and reproductive rights". He is the great unknown unknown and pulls all the strings.

Meantime the tragedy continues to unfold and more and more leading ladies succumb and nobody knows why. This story has continued for 50 or more years and is gathering momentum and is spreading and deepening in age and rapidity of casualties and it's the same background music we hear . . . . "It could be this and it could be that and I'm not so sure about the other but let's wait 'til the next act finishes and then we'll look at the data again". Masterly inactivity. Do nothing and it can only get worse! That's the screenplay and is being enacted to a tee.

TO PILL OR NOT TO PILL?
THAT IS THE QUESTION

Shakespeare can sometimes throw light on life's thorny issues. Hamlet with his malignant brand of ambivalence speaks his thoughts out loud in his soliloquy and questions the meaning of life. He ponders whether it is worthwhile being alive with all the hardships it entails. He concludes that people stay alive because they fear death and fear the known unknown of what is after death:

"For who would bear the Whips and Scorns of time,

the Oppressor's wrong, the proud man's Contumely,

the pangs of despised Love, the Law's delay,

the insolence of Office, and the Spurns that patient merit of the unworthy takes,

when he himself might his Quietus make with bare Bodkin?

Who would Fardels bear, to grunt and sweat under a weary life,

but that the dread of something after death, the undiscovered Country,

from whose bourn no Traveller returns, Puzzles the will" . . . .

There comes a time when the die is cast and the only escape is to face the challenge. The picture of breast cancer morbidity and mortality over the past decades is like the state of Denmark in the tragedy Hamlet. All is a harbinger of doom and decline and the only light on the horizon is being shielded from view. Decisive action is required to pull down the shroud that keeps the truth concealed and allows the tragedy to not only continue but to also gather momentum. The state of breast cancer will get worse if things go on as they have and the nettle of exogenous female hormone exposure (OCs, HRT) is not grasped and seen for what it is:—a major and most insidious and under-rated cause of most, if not all, of the aggressive breast cancer in younger women and also a major contributor to breast cancer in older women.

There is a great swirling of life portrayed in Homer's Odyssey and Iliad with death and war and beauty and valiance painted in surreal colours and sounds. The omens of doom or harbingers of catastrophe abound. In Odyssey 20.61 we see orphan girls abandoned by the gods after their parents were slayed. Aphrodite saw their situation and went to Olympos to ask Zeus the head man to protect these girls until safely married, but while she was doing this the storm-spirits (Harpyiai) snatched them away and delivered them to the ministrations of the detested Erinyes. These latter were 3 avengers of the gods and brought signs and ill omens of the god's displeasure with 5th day disasters or screech-owl appearances that foreshadowed destruction.

These omens and screech-owls are now all too visible in the radiology facilities and side theatres of breast check clinics and hospitals. There is hardly a town or suburb that does not have its own breast check clinic. There is hardly a shop that does not sell pink breast cancer goods. There is hardly a medical journal that does not have articles every other week on new treatment or lab tests for breast cancer. Cancer budgets swell and statistical think tanks crunch numbers after numbers of trends and rises in cancers and especially of breast cancers all over the developed world.

These are the omens of doom. These signs signify a deep seated problem that is ever present in people's minds. It is reminiscent of the tuberculosis epidemics of old that decimated whole populations. It is like the thyroid and cancer peaks that resulted after Chernobyl and the one expected after the nuclear accident last year in Japan. The cholera epidemic on London in 1854 was also such a public health catastrophe. The finding of the cause of this cholera epidemic is instructive in the search for a cause for any epidemic such as the breast cancer one.

The now famous water pump in Broad Street London was the source of the infected water that caused the cholera epidemic there. A local physician John Snow did not accept the popular theory at the time that cholera was due to foul air and instead did his own research and discovered that cholera was in fact a water borne disease and not airborne. This is a good example of someone discounting the prevailing theory of the time which did not somehow explain the localization of the infection, and instead focussed on a novel and challenging suggestion that water and not air was the culprit.

He subsequently went on to eradicate the cholera by stopping the use of water from that pump and by following up on the source of the water which was from a contaminated reservoir. This discovery of Snow's is accredited as the founding event of the science of epidemiology. The process leading to the discovery of the cause in this case was that:

(1) There was a spreading epidemic
(2) The scientific journals and medical thought at the time held that it was a disease spread by air
(3) As of yet the germ basis of illness was not discovered. Dr Snow looked at the big picture and investigated other possibilities that would answer the question of its localization to the Broad

Street area. He matched the area with a series of dots of where people were getting cholera to the water supply of the area and found that it was the Southwark and Vauxhall waterworks which supplied the Broad Street area. He subsequently found this reservoir was situated beside a cesspit infected with cholera.

Epidemiology which studies the patterns, causes and effects of health and disease conditions in defined populations is now an advanced science which began with the work of Dr Snow and others. The patterns of cancer occurrence, type and fluctuation are within its remit and world charts of cancer spread and incidence are publicly available on official cancer websites. Breast cancer really benefits from an epidemiological input given its population and territorial variations. Epidemiology journals publish papers dealing with the possible causes and distribution of breast cancer, but unfortunately like with John Snow another view is needed because the picture is very unclear. Put more correctly another "review" is needed looking like Snow did at the geography of the epidemic and likely sources of the "infection". The following questionnaire is helpful in tackling breast cancer from an epidemiological stand point:

What is the Broad Street water pump for breast cancer?

What is the infected Southwark/Vauxhall cesspit or reservoir for breast cancer?

What is the spread of the cancer; the time frame (when it began, speed of spread, virulence of its mortality)?

What type of persons contract the cancer?

Most importantly, has its contagion spread to new populations and countries?

All these factors give an epidemiological road map for the study of possible causative agents.

Is there any virus, bacterium, inhalant, beverage or food that mirrors this picture?

Is there a substance or medication or tick borne infection that tracks this road map?

Is there a pocket or hot spot that has a much higher level of the cancer (for example cancer clusters are known to occur around nuclear reactors that leak emissions)?

Is it genuinely occurring in the reported numbers or is it a statistical mistake or virtual occurrence?

Has there been a successful cure or treatment that may point to its causation?

Does population screening skew the reported incidence figures?

Is the cancer receding in numbers and spread or getting worse?

What do the experts and official medical and scientific bodies say is the cause and have their targeted interventions based on their assumptions been successful or not?

These are some of the pertinent questions basic to any epidemiological assessment of an illness. Let us take them one by one.

The spread of the breast cancer is a phenomenon which began 50 years ago. Of course it occurred before that but the persistent and increasing scatter of the disease over regions and age groups is documented in cancer data bases covering this time frame. Something happened during those 50 years and is still happening because the pattern is getting worse and has not receded in any of the regions already affected. It is a novel type of cancer in that there are no precedents for its behaviour in any other illness description, because it picks out women and especially young women of all social classes. Take leprosy or tuberculosis for example, these were also of epidemic proportions but they affected definite areas and populations and oftentimes were much more prevalent among the poor and affected all ages and both sexes equally. Breast cancer does not respect social class or population or geographic boundaries. It could be said that like leprosy it has different subtypes but unlike leprosy or tuberculosis no infective agent has been found. It does not behave like an illness with an infective causation because none of the hall marks of infection are present. No bug, no white cell response, no pyrexia, no person to person spread, no common dietary or airborne source, no response to all antiviral or antimicrobial medications.

The type of persons who contract the cancer are disparate as regards age, urban or rural dwelling, and social class—it affects them all. They are not disparate as regards sex since 99% of those affected are female; nor country since those affected are predominantly living in developed countries particularly Western Europe, Japan, Use, Australia etc.; whereas in other less developed areas it's incidence is 80% less than in UK or USA. Thus affluence seems to be a factor. The outlier as regards cancer patterns is that breast cancer is particularly virulent in young women and affects a disproportionately large number of them compared to any other cancer. This is unusual, strange, and noteworthy and stands out a serious clue as to what might be the cause.

More recent data now show that it is beginning to increase in incidence in countries like India, South Africa, South America and the lowest incidences are reported in Africa where figures are also increasing more recently. The WHO website on breast cancer in developing countries is fine but again it does not poleaxe the root cause of the increasing numbers. They sing the same song about diet, obesity, inactivity and "adopting of western types of lifestyle" as their explanation for this spread of cancer. It is really significant that they accept the problem is getting worse, that it does have regional variation, (like big mortality because of late presentation and inadequate treatments) . . . . but the glaring revelation is that breast cancer in underdeveloped regions is now beginning to imitate the 1950s and 60s and 70s incidence pattern it went through in Europe and USA. Epidemiologists must be "excited" about this development because it is another serious clue as to the cause of breast cancer. These patterns and trends are freely available to see on any WHO or official website: just google "breast cancer and developing countries or third world".

Is there another environmental or population vector that could mimic this age and geography spread? Diet has been investigated and it does cause cancer to a degree but would not account for the numbers getting breast cancer. Obesity is important but long exposure to obesity and bad diet and lack of exercise does not apply to young people, because they either are not obese and are not physically inactive and have not been exposed to these cancer inducing behaviours for long enough for breast cancer to result in such big numbers. Alcohol which also is a carcinogen could not account for cancer in the numbers seen in young women, again because not enough of these young people are exposed to enough alcohol for long enough to constitute a cancer risk. They are contributory but by no means are they the root cause. The relative naivety of young women to these risks, at a worse case scenario of 5 to 10 years duration, does not reflect how these carcinogenic risks work. They take longer and in higher doses than young people would have had time to be exposed to them. UV light is not a runner either since it is even more intense in countries with lower breast cancer incidence.

Could it be blood pressure tablets or asthma inhalers? These are more common in Western countries and possibly are now reaching Africa? No. There is no evidence of any medication in the West increasing the occurrence of cancer to epidemic proportions, because it would be known by now, with all the post marketing surveillance and the trials prior to release . . . . well at least this is true for all medications except OCs! Also because then a greater number with cancer would be asthmatic or have blood pressure in which case this would be noticed by doctors and pharmacists. No that's not it. Cigarettes and Khat chewing cause cancer but it is of the lung and oropharynx and besides this is very common in some areas where these cancers abound but not breast cancer.

Finally you look at exogenous female hormone intake as OCs and HRT and find that they mirror the picture, are registered as carcinogens by IARC and do affect females only and do affect younger ones in particular. OCs are now being delivered to third world countries as a part of World Bank dig outs and also as health initiatives by various groups. These increasing trends in OC use can be seen in many websites including the UN Projection discussed by Bongaarts and Johansson in "Future Trends in contraceptive prevalence and method mix in the developing world," published in Studies in Family Planning 2002. To highlight this increasing trend they confirm that the average birth rate per couple in these countries has gone from 6 children per couple to 3 children since 1960. This drop is not all due to OCs but a substantial proportion is and it is projected to rise.

The other population vector that mirrors the breast cancer vector is the declining birth rate. The three mirror images right across the world and time and age spectrum are breast cancer incidence, birth rate decline and increase in contraceptive use. This is epidemiological certainty and it is freely available data to anyone who wants to research it. It is extremely important illness behaviour data. Hot spots for breast cancer are Western Europe and USA and these use more OCs in proportion to the rise in breast cancer incidence numbers.

The numbers of breast cancer cases are true and real and are accepted by all official bodies and if you still doubt the incidence figures look at the treatment and morbidity mortality figures. These are objective numbers of women treated and suffering from and deceased from breast cancer. They are real and not virtual numbers.

What treatment if any cures this cancer? Mastectomy and radiotherapy are definite helps as one would expect. More interesting are the breast cancer specific chemotherapies and the successful ones are anti-oestrogen drugs such as Tamoxifen and Raloxifene, and the aromatase inhibitors which also reduce oestrogen levels. They all, in one way or another, reduce the oestrogen level in the body and reduce the oestrogen assault on the breast. Oestrogen therefore has something to do with breast cancer. There are oestrogen receptors in breast tissue, and not surprisingly it is in young women with these very oestrogen receptor sensitive breast cells that the majority of cases of advanced aggressive breast cancer occurs.

Screening for breast cancer is an important adjunct in management of a population at risk and there is controversy over how low should you go before biopsy, prophylactic chemotherapy, surgery etc. What is independent of screening however, is the prevalence of real metastatic and spreading cancer, and this is increasing and has increased by up to 70% in UK, as the official cancer site testifies—as have breast cancer deaths and numbers in treatment. Screening may and often does catch it early but the big numbers (metastatic cancer and deaths) are still solid and increasing. The hard core aggressive cancer and the morbidity and mortality figures are also increasing despite nationwide screening. The breast cancer epidemic is also increasing in developing countries where there is no screening.

The occurrence of the disease has nowhere receded or gone away in any country where it occurred. It is not abating but getting steadily worse in intensity in virulence and in geographic spread. (All the facts referenced in these last paragraphs are referenced in other parts of this monograph but have not been repeated again here to allow the flow of the discussion).

What interventions have the experts conducted and what were they and what were the results? Experts advise diet, good BMI (body mass index) figures, exercise, moderate alcohol, no cigarettes, and regular self breast checking for lumps etc. They recommend tamoxifen or prophylactic mastectomy in high risk women (BRCA 1and 2 gene mutation, strong family history, previous breast cancer). In other words good behaviours recommended for avoiding any type of cancer and also specific anti-oestrogens for high risk breast cancer. The epidemic is getting worse despite these interventions and advice.

REFLECTIONS WITH FURTHER EVIDENCE

More analogies from Homer's Odyssey

It could well be said that language hasn't been invented yet to describe the horrors of war, the pangs of unrequited love or the ecstasy of delight. Words and literature are firstly communication and after that a form of art which is also a form of more sublime or abstract communication.

Sometimes things are so bad that you cannot even think of them not to mind talk about them. When two super powers (prime ministers, presidents, kings) meet, and both are only but too keenly aware of the burning issues they may have to discuss, they sometimes may not even allude or mention them in conversation. Be convinced however that the burning issue really is the topic and it is the body language and voice intonation and eye contact that reveal the true sub text and the real point of the meeting. They say that when the Secretary of State of the US met the Finance minister of Japan they spoke mainly about their interest in Orchids. When the Irish golfer Padraigh Harrington was struggling in the 3ʳᵈ round of the PGA Championship he rang his psychologist who said "drink more water". He did and won. So words are useful but often don't show the charge on them. Who is saying what to whom and when? Circumstance, personalities involved and the content of what is said and how it is said and to whom are all important, and body language is much more powerful than words most of the time. This applies very much to the breast cancer language used by those who set the agenda and who lead the public and scientific debate. Sometimes the unspoken words are the key communication. A laid back laissez faire attitude to breast cancer causation in the epicentre of a breast cancer storm that is growing is definitely bizarre. Someone somewhere is asleep at the job or has jammed the lines. The screech-owls are now exhausted with their feet up in the air and the last few omens are petering out. What more warning do they need? An out break of aggressive breast cancer in a herd of cows grazing on lands irrigated by effluent from a contraceptive manufacturing plant for example? Even that would be explained away or suppressed.

How about this omen. In 2009 a study of triple negative breast cancer (TNBC) in women under 45 years, a very aggressive type of cancer with a high mortality was published in the well known journal—Cancer Epidemiol Biomarkers Prev 2009. The authors reported that recent users of the pill within the last 1 to 5 years multiply their risk of TNBC by 4.2 times. Women who started using the pill before age 18 multiply their risk of TNBC by 3.7 times. This report was effectively ignored and no mainstream journalist covered it except the Chicago Tribune. This is what has been a repetitive response to good hard data on breast cancer causation. The "it never happened, we never heard that, you better check your facts", response. Those that are forced to comment offer banalities such as "we see that, but lets wait for better data", and what do you know, if "better data" is needed it can be obtained. For example a metanalysis with all kinds of data included could be grandstanded and the TNBC study is then swallowed up in this "bigger picture". Look at most of the metanalyses on this topic to see what has happened. The metanalysis by Chris Kahlenborn showing a 44% increase in breast cancer for women, who started the pill before their first pregnancy, was completely ignored by the mainstream press even though it was published in The Mayo Clinic Proceedings journal and press releases were issued to all major media outlets.

Another screeching owl flew over and smashed into a wall with the media hype "celebrating" the 50th anniversary of the pill in 2010. All the big guns were out with innocuous articles about the past, its rubberstamping by the FDA in 1960 . . . . was it May 9th Mother's Day or was it June 23rd? . . . type of stuff. The Times UK, The New York Times, Washington Post, Time magazine all did their catwalk and no smell of sulphur and no roses for the deceased—care of the pill. This was another great feather in the cap of those who say the pill is safe. The Planned Parenthood site did admit that 19% of women between the ages of 15 and 44 use the pill, (and I say it comes as no surprise that many of them get aggressive breast cancer). The latter they do not say.

Type "breast cancer" into the Planned Parenthood site, and up come lists for screening for breast cancer etc. and how to detect it early. Most people would have expected a walk through the: "How not to get breast cancer," portfolio. No, just do this if you've got it and we are here to help and serve you. "Thank you" you may say "and when do I start screening, or screaming, is the more appropriate word?" Well what do you expect from one of the major promoters of birth control and oral contraception? It's like going into a garage when your new car breaks down and they tell you "sorry we don't do breakdowns if you read the brochure carefully you will see that we sell cars only and if you don't get that we can have you removed. We sold the car it's your problem if it breaks down. See to it yourself." They are legally covered, it says it in the brochure, and it's your problem. "We can screen it for malfunctions or signs of possible future breakdown and that is $500 for a basic check . . . . alternatively we can hook you up to the computer diagnostics for $235."

The message is clear. This web site does not say it but it is each woman's free and responsible choice to pill or not to pill and take the consequences. At this stage more than 50 years on and after millions of new breast cancers and deaths at all too young ages which surprisingly mirror OC usage patterns, the die is cast. Take it at your peril. Shakespeare again advises with his speech from Brutus in Julius Caesar:

"There is a tide in the affairs of men which taken at the flood leads on to fortune;
Omitted all the voyage of their life is bound in shallows and in miseries.

On such a full sea are we now afloat, and we must take the current when it serves, or lose our ventures."

Taken in the present context it points to a full tide of good research by reputable authors pointing to real and present danger of breast cancer from OCs; and armed with this information and the statistics of new breast cancer cases and breast cancer deaths over 35 years or more; and observing it's present spread to new regions following the introduction of OCs there; what more is there to say? The IARC have graded OCs as a number 1 carcinogen and The World Health Organisation categorise it up there with cigarettes and other well established cancer causing agents. These facts are either ignored and forgotten about which is what is happening; or else, they are acted upon and this action will lead on to fortune and the stemming of the breast cancer scourge. This taking the tide in the affairs of men at the flood will not be from above down. No official body or prestigious journal or political heavyweight will shout stop and have the power to turn the tide. It will be as always in human rights issues a grassroots bottom up slowly growing and eventually powerful will of the people. Breast cancer is happening, it's advancing, and it's being allowed to progress. Why? The strongest bias and obstacle to anything is when you don't want something to be true or that you see it as a threat to your dearest project.

This type of bias is practically insurmountable when it is arising from a deeply entrenched and held view. This is the case with the pill. It is more than a pill. It is more than dollars. IT IS A PHILOSOPHICAL WORLDVIEW. It is "I want it and I want it now and to hell with the consequences". The problem with this is that delusions are contagious and follie a deux, a troix, a milliones is happening i.e mass hysteria or delusion. The control over reproduction has gone viral and it is untenable for decades now to even think about having more than the regulatory 2.1 children. This has cost millions of women's lives from the side effects of the pill and other birth control methods. The powers in control do not accept this and they deny, ignore, cover up, air brush and stamp out any opposing voices. They can do this because they have the money, the contacts the media and the politicians. This is the real reason behind this breast cancer disaster. People who know the dangers are actively pushing OCs as a life choice and a way of living, and nature says no, and reacts with breast cancer and other side effects of exposure to too much female hormones.

CONCLUSIONS

This is a terrible story, a terrible illness and it will have a terrible ending unless the present trend of tit for tat conflicting research reports is ended. This guerrilla warfare in the medical literature is self perpetuating and has a life of its own. It is a virtual reality sustained by bias, vested interest, and statistical and publishing spin to some degree. In the midst of the fog a sometimes glimmer of simple truth can be seen in transparent well conducted and independent studies.

These lines have tried to depict an illness that has grown over 50 or so years, has and is advancing and has the potential to get much worse. The broad strokes and sometimes outrageous expression used here have been employed to refresh, refocus, and try to put the picture in a graphic and knife edge focus. This in turn may stimulate someone somewhere to get an insight or reaction or inspiration to do something about it, or to get a new approach that may cut this epidemic to the quick. Women are the main victims but also their loved ones and our sincerest sympathies go to them. If the hypothesis advanced here is incorrect let it be disproved simply and transparently. It is up to the naysayers to show why they say it is wrong so that the simplest of us can see and acknowledge it. Unfortunately it is not wrong but obvious and true and it has been constantly denied, ignored and contradicted for over 35 years. The recent good new data some of which has been presented here is a great opportunity to stop the progression of breast cancer now and bring closure to this sad epidemic. If this opportunity is missed it may not happen again for another 25 years in which case swards of new women, countries and populations will have been affected.

This is not a quest for scientific discovery as much as a plea to arrest the devastation of a spreading cancer. The knowledge base and treatments for all types of cancers have grown exponentially over the recent decades. Illnesses such as tuberculosis and HIV and even mental illness have seen enormous advances in treatment, diagnosis, prognosis and partial eradication. Why cannot the same happen with breast cancer? It can, but the obvious cause must not be ignored. Those who direct the breast cancer endeavour and funnel funding to other secondary fields to the neglect of the primary concern of causation and prevention, are doing what they consider their jobs. The overarching reality however of cancer progression and spread is thus ignored or evokes the response "we have looked at that before and others have and the studies show OCs don't really cause much breast cancer". Everyone knows breast cancer is all too common especially in young women, and evidence from trends in research shows they accept it as fact of life, and women's Pink Ribbon groups seem to accept it, and all "the King's horses and all the King's men." There needs to be a vocal group that says "Hey wait a minute let's look at that again, there is something seriously wrong in this whole business. Breast cancer is getting out of control and the obvious cause is being said not to cause it . . . . then what is causing it? They must have gotten it wrong and we'd have better find out as soon as possible."

The social and geo political narrative of this cancer and the enormous tail it is dragging behind it in the form of women's rights, control of fertility, meaning of motherhood and lobby group influences and various other interested parties, make this much more complicated than a simple quest to elucidate the cause of an illness. It is also a battle of world views and philosophical understanding. This explains possibly why it has taken so long to get a clue to its causation and why a simple statement on the genuine and real risk of exogenous female hormones has not been forth coming from the medical and cancer establishments.

The enormous societal changes that have happened in the developed world in the past century as regards the roles of women and men and family were a work in progress and a result of the changes occurring in the working environment with and as a result of the industrial revolution. These changes were also the result of the progressive maturing of the male-female-family-society dynamic into a level playing field where each human being has equal rights and their natural differences (male, female child, handicapped, ill or healthy etc.) are respected and supported by society. The pill and birth control occurred by coincidence at the same time but were not the cause or root of the good societal transformation that was happening. To a large extent proponents of birth control hijacked the changes and laid the results of all the societal changes at their own door. This is and was a travesty of truth and justice and fuller discussion of this topic is for another forum.

Breast cancer is a sign of something deeper in the fabric of modern western culture. It is one of the bad side effects of the radical changes that have occurred in society. It is a societal cancer to some extent and when this is acknowledged and steps are taken to reverse the trend of widespread OC birth control then the incidence of breast cancer will recede.